CO ABW 726

Innovation in Health Policy and Service Delivery

PUBLICATION OF THE SCIENCE CENTER BERLIN
Volume 34

Innovation in Health Policy and Service Delivery

A Cross-National Perspective

Research on Service Delivery
Volume III

Edited by
Christa Altenstetter
Queens College and
The City University of New York

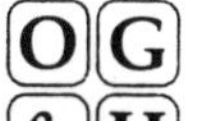
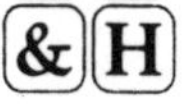
Oelgeschlager, Gunn & Hain, *Publishers,* Inc.
Cambridge, Massachusetts

Verlag Anton Hain • Königstein/Ts.

International Standard Book Number: 0-89946-078-x (U.S.A.)
ISBN 3-445-121270-2 (Germany)

Library of Congress Catalog Card Number: 80-39617

Printed in West Germany

Library of Congress Cataloging in Publication Data
Main entry under title:

Innovation in health policy and service delivery.

Includes index.
1. Medical policy–Congresses. 2. Medical innovations –Congresses. 3. Health services administration–Congresses. 4. Medical care–Cross-cultural studies–Congresses. I. Altenstetter, Christa. [DNLM: 1. Health policy. 2. Delivery of health care. W 84.1 I58]
RA2.I56 362.1′068 80-39617
ISBN 0-89946-078-x

Contents

Foreword

This is the third publication of the Science Center Berlin on research on service delivery. It is one of the Science Center's main tasks to venture into new research fields relating to urgent social and political problems. Public services are a major problem area. In the Federal Republic of Germany, as in other Western countries, the proportion of the service industries in the labor force as well as in the GNP is steadily increasing. Accordingly, the expansion of the service sector is becoming more and more subject to criticism and analysis. The criticism is primarily directed at the quantitative and qualitative expansion of services and the financial and personal resources they require. However, these evident trends must be interpreted in the wider context of social changes in highly industrialized countries. A report of the Organization for Economic Cooperation and Development (OECD), *Innovations in the Social Services,* took up this problem and encouraged research in the field.

Within the framework of the research program of the International Institute of Management at the Science Center Berlin, a number of activities were initiated in the past few years in the problem area of "service delivery." They soon went beyond the scope of single projects and became a research program in their own right. The scientists involved in these projects decided to unite their efforts with researchers at the University of Bielefeld working in the same field; together, they formulated an integrated research program covering problems of health services, legal services, and social services.

As part of the initial research and stimulated by the abovementioned OECD report, the Science Center held, in cooperation with the OECD, an international conference on "Innovations in Service Delivery" in the summer of 1978. I am very pleased to include these conference proceedings in our publication series; the discussion and results of this conference demonstrate the relevance of the approaches developed at the Science Center in the research field of service delivery.

Needless to say, the responsibility for the data, results and conclusions presented rests solely with the authors.

Helmut G. Meier
Secretary General
1974–1979
Science Center Berlin

Chapter 1

Introduction

Christa Altenstetter

The current popularity of innovation suggests a political as well as a common-sense appeal, but its meaning is unclear. Being part of the repertoire of national political and administrative elites, innovation is frequently invoked. Indeed, much of the talk about innovation and the demand for its implementation fall into the category of political window dressing. An inverse relationship seems to exist between the frequency and the intensity of exhortations to innovate—such as "creative innovation," "creative potential," "innovative change"—and our lack of knowledge, at least in the fields of health and social policy, about the causes of or conditions that conduce to substantial and substantive innovation in specific rather than in general terms. The term *innovative technology(ies)* seems to compound the confusion. The term *technology* signals a shorthand way of referring to fundamentally different things. Technology is frequently equated with hardware and suggests uniformity and homogeneity, hence manageability and malleability, and the application of highly sophisticated and specialized tools. The mastery of techniques seems to be the essential prerequisite for the application and the implementation of technology. But this indiscriminate use of the term *innovative technology(ies)* is misleading. The bulk of technologies politicians and administrative officials speak of are clearly of a political nature.

In looking at technology and innovation from a multidisciplinary and cross-national vantage point, additional conceptual distinctions and values emerge. Despite the appearance of a homogeneous language that transcends national and linguistic boundaries, considerable differences exist because people who live in different political and cultural environments attribute to one and the same concept different activities as well as methodological tools, although scholars from these diverse settings would probably be able to agree about the abstract definitions of these terms.

What we know that may be considered systematic and scientific knowledge about the diffusion and the adoption of innovation, and adaptive behavior, stems largely from economic and organizational studies conducted in the private sector on industrial products (including drugs, medical equipment, and medical hardware technology). Another body of literature addresses innovations in the delivery of services and local health agencies as well as the impact of medical technology on the treatment of patients/clients. This literature is primarily microorganizational and sociological. Studies about innovation and implementation in public organizations are receiving increased attention. And, finally, the literature that treats innovation as an expression of dynamic interaction patterns and communication networks or that treats innovation as a reflection of the political process of mutual adjustment offers a fruitful framework for the study of innovation and technology. But cross-national and single-country studies about the innovation of health policies, public or private organizations in the health field, and service delivery are scarce, especially those that differentiate between problems associated with the implementation of medical care in contrast to health care policies.

If innovation means "the introduction of something new, a new idea, method, or device," and if to innovate means "to introduce something new and to make changes," then we may be able to agree about what innovation is *not.* The introduction of change has always required social, behavioral, and organizational adaptation that has not always been forthcoming. If budget constraints, limited economic growth, limited capabilities for effecting change, and largely unknown returns from society's financial and human investments summarize the main causes of today's increased demands for innovation, then we should remember that such circumstances have occurred in the history of many countries, and in some countries more than once. Social conflicts over power, resources, the control of techniques, and opposition to a shift of powerholders seem to denote what historical development is all about.

What distinguishes yesterday's innovations from today's are the conditions under which they take place, the scale and the complexity of the kinds of problems that face innovators today, and the considerable division of tasks that characterizes political and administrative management. But what seems equally crucial is the fact that in some areas of health, as in other social policy areas, responding to pressures might have generated too many changes too soon to record the impact of individual changes. On the other hand, hardly any change has taken place in other areas. We may, indeed, raise the question: Does the modern problem really involve the lack of proposals for change, or are we confronted with a kind of innovation overload with which service organizations and lower-level public or quasi-public organizations in the health field have to cope? This problem is intensified when inconsistent decisions are made.

Although there is clarity in the diagnosis of the problems associated with innovation, the magnitude of these problems, and the shifting role and capabilities of the governmental sector in industrial nations, there is much less consensus in the proposed remedies. The Report on Innovation for Policies in the Public Services of the Organization of Economic Cooperation and Development (OECD) in 1977 summarized these generalizations:

Innovation

1. Innovation in services increasingly focuses on systems.
2. Innovation depends on flexibility.
3. The uncertainty about consequences and about the assumption of risks is an important determinant of innovation.
4. Innovation has increasingly become a function of complex knowledge and its application.
5. Innovation depends on the integration of diverse actions.
6. Technological innovation remains of major importance; however, its limitations have aroused considerable concern.
7. Innovation in services increasingly depends on the achievement of consensus.
8. Many innovations appear to be incremental in nature.
9. Experiment as innovation offers a promising approach to service delivery.
10. Innovation requires personal incentives.

The Problem

Public-Sector Services

1. Services have expanded in number and in kind in response to the growth of governmental responsibility for public welfare.
2. Public-sector services are increasingly confronted with problems of a challenging nature.

3. Services depend on large and complex infrastructures.
4. Interaction among services has compounded the difficulties of delivering services.
5. The formal evaluation of many public-sector services has become increasingly important.
6. Service benefits are increasingly compromised by factors once considered beyond the scope of service concern.
7. Significant changes in the relationships between professional, expert authorities and the public have affected service delivery.

Government

1. Government has assumed the major institutional responsibility for providing services in the public interest.
2. The growth in governmental responsibilities has been accompanied by the growing incidence of difficulties in resolving practical service issues.
3. Public concern with the processes and goals of service delivery is reflected in the changed mode of government operations.
4. The structure, organization, and personnel of government play major roles in delivering services.
5. The growth of governmental authority and activity has led to a reduction in the involvement of the private sector in the delivery of services.
6. The capability of government to continue to act effectively is threatened by the expansion of its responsibilities.

This report inspired the convening of an international conference in Berlin on June 13–16, 1978, which was sponsored jointly by the Organisation for Economic Co-operation and Development (OECD) and the Science Center Berlin (Wissenchaftszentrum Berlin). Scholars from eight countries and different disciplinary backgrounds gathered to discuss some propositions in the context of innovations in health and medical care policies and in the delivery of health and medical services. Needless to say, this meeting could not address all aspects of innovation and medical technology. Those aspects that were addressed constitute only a first treatment of the subject. Freed from the burden of having to pronounce success when more realistic assessments of recent policies and innovations in the health sector suggest modest performance or, in the worst case, failure, the meeting in Berlin sought to develop generalizations by focusing on the historical, economic, political, and sociological factors that have produced the present difficulties in an effort to understand the nature of these problems and constraints before prescribing a new dosage of innovations. The cases presented at the Berlin meeting expanded the perspective of the OECD report, which focused on the learning ability and adaptive capacity of the public-service sector from the vantage point of those responsible for managing the services and applying strategies available to them.

Cases on innovation and targets of change ranged from innovations in policy, to financial and organizational procedures, to social and human innovations, and to learning capabilities (personal and institutional). A first group of cases, in Part I, deals with the problems of policymaking in the field of health and medical care, reflecting the heterogeneous nature of the services provided, the difficulty of measuring outputs in any meaningful way, and the fact that the organization of service delivery is the product of social and political processes and conditioning, in sharp contrast to industry.

Another group of cases—in Part II—addresses the problems posed by medical technology in the practice of medicine: problems of definition, perception, development, diffusion, adoption, use and abuse, and, finally the evaluation and the abandonment of medical technology. These cases fall into two distinct categories. The first includes a critical examination of these problems at the societal and macro policymaking levels; the second involves a study of these problems at the level of applying medical technology to diagnosis, treatment, and different kinds of caring for and about patients.

The final group of cases (Part III) deals with specific examples of the organization of service delivery and intergovernmental and interorganizational relations. The subject ranges from labor-union innovations in workers' medicine as an alternative to state-interventionist strategies, to problems of coordinating and integrating health services with related social services, to innovations in the relationship of central to local governments and central institutions to local institutions.

Although cases, single and multicountry alike, are limited in the generalizability of their findings, they constitute valuable and rich laboratories for discovering fertile ground for comparative analysis and testing hunches about interrelated factors that explain unique and general elements in innovation, innovation targets, agents of change, and mechanisms of change. Because different perspectives about the same problem can be brought to bear on explanations, the value of cases is enhanced by an interdisciplinary approach. But explanations also become more complex. Real-life experiences with innovation in medical care and health policy and service delivery in Sweden, Finland, England, the Netherlands, France, the Federal Republic of Germany, Italy, the United States, and Canada testify to the infinite variety of reality and explain success, failure, modest performance, and obstacles to recent public interventions mandated by law or tried out voluntarily. For example, one country pursued a centralist strategy, ignoring long-standing traditions of local autonomy and decentralization. These traditional forces counteracted implementation. Learning from experience, the decision was made to move in the direction of decentralization. This reversal may indeed testify to the function of the policy cycle through feedback, but we are not sure. In other countries, the centralization of decision making seems to be progressing.

In short, what is an appropriate and applicable solution in one country may not be so in another. Why? Some traditional forces counteract centralization, and some counteract decentralization, such as the tradition of centralization in politics, administration, and financing that characterizes health policymaking and administration in most European countries. How can countries revert from this tradition of bureaucratic centralism and the domination of the center over the periphery to more decentralized approaches? Cultural behavior and the traditions of these political systems seem to have provided some answers. But these answers differ from country to country and from clusters of countries to others.

Case materials help identify the similarities and dissimilarities of phenomena across societies. They also help identify the uniqueness of the health and medical-care sectors when compared to other services sectors because health and medical-care services are expensive *and* primarily manpower intensive and technology intensive. Another feature characterizes authority and responsibility in the field of health in most countries: Authority and responsibility are delegated to a considerable degree to private, quasi-public, or other intermediate agencies. The extent of this delegation is quite striking when compared to that which obtains in other policy fields. In addition, the beliefs of professionals and of the public in many countries seem to converge on similar preferences. Popular beliefs affirm that "the best practice is the one with the newest medical technology"—in most cases, the most expensive. From the vantage point of the medical profession, this popular demand can be met only "when the best medical care that can be given is technically possible."

One impression emerges from the cases and from the lively exchange of ideas that occurred at the meeting in Berlin. As is manifest in the political arenas in most countries, much of the concern reflected in the OECD report and voiced at the international meeting centered on the economic costs of high medical technology. There seems to be a fascination with the subject that declines or increases according to the geographic provenance of analysts and participants. Admittedly, problems of costs and controls related to high-cost medical technology are serious, but with the political will to act, they can be solved. The real and long-term issues in the sector of services are political problems: conflicts resulting from a shift in power relationships and a shift in policy, mechanisms for implementation, regulatory interventions, and organizational innovations that emanate from a professionally dominated care system to innovations that constructively use other service providers. These and the following issues seem to deserve more attention than they have received.

The rise of highly skilled medical professionals and the significance of the bureaucracy(ies) in structuring and implementing policy alternatives have been the subject of much writing in the social sciences. Lately it has become fashionable in the Western world to criticize "professionalism" and to point out the excessive amount of "bureaucratization" that characterizes many aspects of modern life. Without discounting the fact that the demand for deprofessionalization and debureaucratization may belong to the current rhetoric, this criticism, which, for quite different reasons, comes from all poles of the political spectrum, is largely justified. Looking at the unequal distribution of social and economic power and the rewards that relate to prestige, status, and the positions of both bureaucrats and professionals when compared to other socioeconomic groups in society, or in looking at the decreasing space for private initiatives and prerogatives not regulated by the state, such complaints are warranted. However, they also articulate global and simplistic notions that completely ignore the historical record and the roles played by professional and bureaucratic groups as crucial agents of change at different periods of social and political transformations.

The contributions that these two groups have made as agents of change or as obstructors of change differ considerably from country to country. There will be great variations in the change potential of these two groups in the future. How does one explain the differences in health and medical care systems across societies? Are the decisions made by policymakers the ultimate ones? Or does our explanation need to take into consideration the parts played by these two groups that have been placed at important decision-making points not only within the professional and bureaucratic infrastructures but also within the political-administrative system?

Could reforms have succeeded without the sustained political support given by these two groups? The historical record and cross-national experiences give clear answers. For major reforms to be institutionalized, changes need the support of these two groups. Countries vary greatly in the extent to which they have used health professionals other than physicians. In this case, too, it seems that changes in service delivery and care evolved from *within* the respective professions.

PART I

Macro Health Policies: Culture and Health, Distribution of Care, Allocating Resources

After reviewing health decisions that were formulated and adopted by governments over the last decade, Jean de Kervasdoué critically examines why certain issues were never entered on agendas for decision making and why those that were seem to have converged across societies in terms of two main themes: (a) the pursuit of equality issues, and (b) the imposition of control instruments over the practice of medical care inside and outside hospitals. From the perspective of organization theory, Jean de Kervasdoué raises questions concerning the appropriateness of governmental responses and the compatibility of selected control instruments with the objectives of health policy and medical practice. By drawing on comparative studies about aspects of European and American health-care systems, a number of theoretical questions are formulated that are dealt with more extensively in subsequent cases in this volume. These questions relate to performance criteria, the determinants of the practice of medicine and medical behavior, remuneration systems, the allocation of medical resources in the treatment of patients, and the role of policymakers in solving or exacerbating some of the problems in the health field.

Within this theoretical framework, two cases explore specific strategies using a change in financing as a vehicle for innovation. The dominant political economy and the insitutional and financial characteristics of the American health-care system seem to have influenced the outcome of the cases. Theodore R. Marmor and James A. Morone examine the objectives of governmental intervention in initiating service arrangements as an alternative to the dominant mode of delivering and financing medical services. They also assess the different kinds of impacts of what seemed to be a genuine organizational and financial innovation. Thomas W. Bice describes the origin, the objectives, and the mechanisms of regulatory controls in the American hospital sector that were mandated by law in the hope of curtailing health-cost inflation. Reporting on earlier findings of a nationwide study, he examines the impact of regulatory controls on hospital-investment behavior and per capita health-care costs during 1968–1972.

Chapter 2

Are Health Policies Adapted to the Practice of Medical Care?

Jean de Kervasdoué

The growing importance of expenses for health in developing countries as well as the growing awareness of disparities in the distribution of and access to care have led governments in those countries, especially during the last ten years, to intervene more directly in matters of health care. In the policies that have been developed, reference is usually made to at least one if not both of the following concepts: equality and control.

Equality of access to care is not a new concept. The first insurance programs, designed to compensate for inequalities in income, were established more than fifty years ago. The limitations of access to care based on patient income have been disappearing little by little in most countries and for most kinds of care. Furthermore, equality has come to mean more than ensuring that all individuals, regardless of income, can use the health system. It also means geographic equality, that is, the equal availability of medical care. In practice, equality in the second sense has come to mean the establishment of ratios, such as the number of hospital beds per thousand inhabitants, or various methods designed to encourage doctors to locate in areas where medical care is relatively scarce.

The use of the word *control* is more recent but is becoming more frequent. At first, the concept of control was applied primarily to costs. To control costs, attempts were made to limit the supply of medical personnel, which was limited in other respects for monopolistic reasons (Stephan, 1978), the supply of equipment (hospital beds, scanners, radiological equipment), and the supply of new drugs.

Methods of management developed and applied in industry were also introduced. In such instances the term *control* was used in the sense of managerial control, a concept underlying cost-benefit analyses and cost-effectiveness studies. Then in the early 1970s the word *quality* became associated with the word *control.* The creation, in October 1972, of PSROs (Professional Standard Review Organization) in the United States represented the first important attempt to introduce quality control into the health arena. The objective of the PSROs was to establish a process whereby doctors would define quality criteria on an illness-by-illness basis. They also involved the establishment of rules for the use of equipment because it had been shown that equality of health care is related to the rate of use and that underuse results in significantly lower quality.

In this chapter we will demonstrate that the control of quality, the control of care, equality of access, and equality of distribution are contradictory objectives. We will then examine the results of different concrete measures taken in various European countries with respect to the quality of care, the geographic distribution of equipment and medical personnel, and health costs.

To begin to understand those problems in health, it is necessary, first, to consider the practical tools that are available to managers and politicians, especially control procedures. It is necessary to understand how those tools limit and even distort the practice of medicine and why they generally do not produce the intended consequences. Certain countries, of course, are succeeding and others will succeed in maintaining for a short period of time a certain stability in health costs by introducing, for example, rationing procedures. But it is unlikely that those solutions will last long for reasons that relate to the difference between medical technology and control techniques.

The basic argument of this chapter begins with a discussion of different control systems. Particular attention will be paid to the relationship between techniques designed to achieve the goals of organized human activity and the methods developed to control those techniques. There is a considerable gap between the nature of a task and the tools available to accomplish it. In the case of medicine, those tools actually transform the nature of this activity and lead to a system that is hierarchical, unfair, and expensive. The analysis will show how political/administrative rules are used by various interest groups (health professionals, administrators, the biomedical industry, and others) and how public support enables groups in power to strengthen their positions.[1]

Before examining more closely the production of health—or, perhaps more precisely, the medical system—it is necessary to place this organized activity into a larger context.

1. TECHNOLOGY AND CONTROL

Modern management methods (a synonym for control) that are taught in business schools were developed in industrial firms. In that kind of organization, one can often link means and ends in a direct way, or, in the language of the economists, one can define a production function. Methods are thus based on a mechanistic conception of organizations and society.[2] To produce an automobile or a washing machine, it is known how many men, how many tons of steel, and how many electric circuits are needed. The task involves optimizing the number of hours, men, and raw material per unit of production. Such optimization is called moving toward maximal efficiency. Such measures can be useful indicators, even though it has been shown that they are not necessarily sufficient on a long-term basis (the difference between effectiveness and efficiency).

But an organization is not merely an empty shell, as certain structuralists would lead us to believe, or simply a production function, as certain economists would have us believe. As we indicated in previous work (de Kervasdoué and Kimberly, 1978), an organization can only be understood if one takes into account the strategies of various groups for whom it is potentially valuable, whether those groups represent members of the organization or take an economic, a political, or even a symbolic interest in the organization.

In a metaphoric sense, groups develop various game plans that they implement on the playing field. The analogue of the playing field is technology,[3] which, when used in the sense intended here, means not only the combination of tools and knowledge that leads to certain consequences but also the organizational norms that are associated with it. Technology cannot be separated from the results of its application. On the other hand, some techniques are more easily formalized than others, that is, broken down into their basic components, and some, when applied, lead to results that are more measurable than others. Both the extent to which a technology can be formalized and the ability to measure the results of its application are important factors in the strategies of different groups. But because the results of all technologies are not equally measurable, the strategies of different groups that have varying interests in particular technologies will vary from one case to the next.

1.1. Results Are More or Less Measurable

Two relatively simple indexes can be used to measure the output of a firm producing electricity—the number of kilowatt hours produced and the average cost per kilowatt hour. However, it is more difficult to evaluate the extent to which the objectives of a research center or of the Catholic church have been attained. Two words and/or two sets of numbers certainly would not be sufficient. Even the appropriate dimensions of analysis would be subject to debate, to say nothing of the way in which measures could be operationalized. Between these two extremes, there is an infinite number of possibilities. There can be multiple criteria, some of which are immeasurable quantitatively, that is, on a cardinal scale, and others that are only qualitatively estimable, that is, on a nominal scale. There can be criteria that relate to means and criteria that relate to results or only one and not the other. To keep the argument simple, only the extreme cases are considered here.

1.2. The Technology Is More or Less Susceptible to Formalization

Since the beginning of the century, under the influence of Taylorism, the skills of various professions have been supplanted by repetitive and formalized processes; however, there are still many patterns of human activities that have not yet reached the stage at which every ten-thousandth of an hour on the assembly line is programmed and nothing is left to chance. The hand of the sculptor has not yet been programmed. The best way to transmit knowledge is not known. Nor is the manner in which a doctor makes his diagnosis formalized. It is not known how many people and how much money it takes to make a "good" film.[4]

Simply because the results of technology can be evaluated in some terms (that is, a film might have been viewed by ten of fifty thousand people) does not mean that the technology is potentially susceptible to formalization.

These two dimensions lead us to four ideal-typical categories; see Figure 2.1.

Logically there should be no organizations listed in cells 3 and 4. Why are some organizations found there? Why are some technologies formalized, although potentially they are not susceptible to formalization? To answer these questions, it is necessary to examine what we call the paradox of bureaucratization.[5]

The paradox of bureaucratization takes the form of the following question: Why are the most highly formalized, most rigid organizations found in areas that are the least susceptible to formalization?

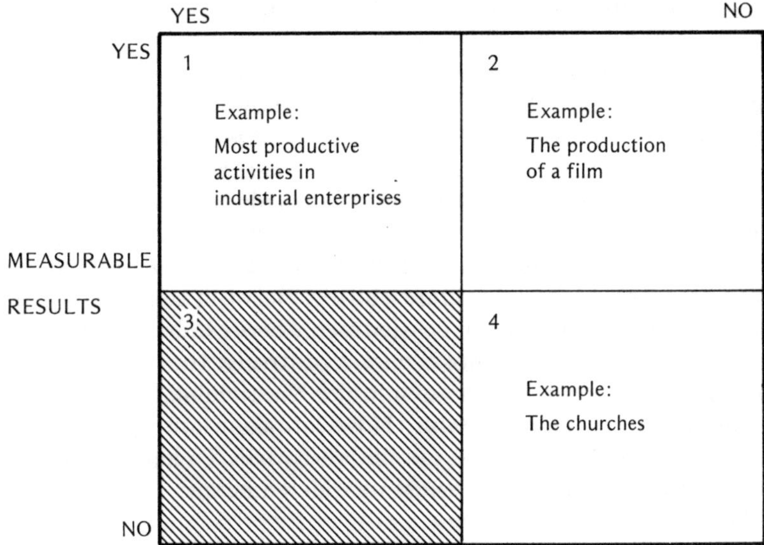

Figure 2.1. Formalizable technology.

This paradox can be explained, at least in part, by reference to the entrepreneurial theory of organizations formulated by Becker and Gordon (1966). According to them, an organization is created by an owner in order to take advantage of either the division of labor or the sharing of resources. Unfortunately for the owner—whose objectives can be either economic or moral—it is necessary to hire employees who may subsequently usurp the resources of the organization, that is, they may use the means granted them by the owner to achieve their own personal objectives, not those of the owner. The ease with which the owner's resources may be usurped depends on the type of organization, as defined in Figure 2.1. When goals are measurable and the technology is known and programmed, the owner can ascertain the extent to which his goals are being achieved and can also determine the contribution of each person at each stage in the production process. The dangers of usurpation are thus reduced to an absolute minimum, and the means of control are simple. Control is ensured if rules and procedures defining the production process are followed.[6] The owner will thus try to approximate this ideal insofar as possible and will try to move his organization toward cell 1.

The problem, of course, is how to proceed when the technology is not objectively programmable and has not been perfected. In such cases, the justification for a particular technology is no longer rooted in demonstrable efficiency but in some cultural arena. When the utility of a technology cannot be demonstrated in a straightforward analysis of its efficacy, other forms of validation, deriving, for example, from moral or religious values, may be substituted. In such cases, the organization performs a social role that is more ritual than rational in the Weberian sense and leads to Figure 2.2.

In this way the technology of psychiatric hospitals has existed as a function of the a priori definition of the mentally ill (Perrow, 1966); schools have developed and survived without any real proof of the efficacy of the dominant pedagogical technology in comparison to alternative but culturally unthinkable technologies; the most rigid bureaucracies (such as social welfare, the prevention of delinquency, and so on) exist in areas in which alternative technologies exist but the merits of the technology in use have not been demonstrated firmly. The most rigid bureaucracies exist in those areas in which the technology is cultural and the outcomes are unmeasurable. How can the merits of a particular change be assessed if there is no consensus about what should change and how the impact of the change should be measured?

The organizational consequences of a given technology are, among others, a hierarchy, a division of labor, and a reward system. The employees of an organization decide to participate (March and Simon, 1958) for reasons that do not need to be made explicit in this paper. But it can be said that they are sensitive to any change that could threaten

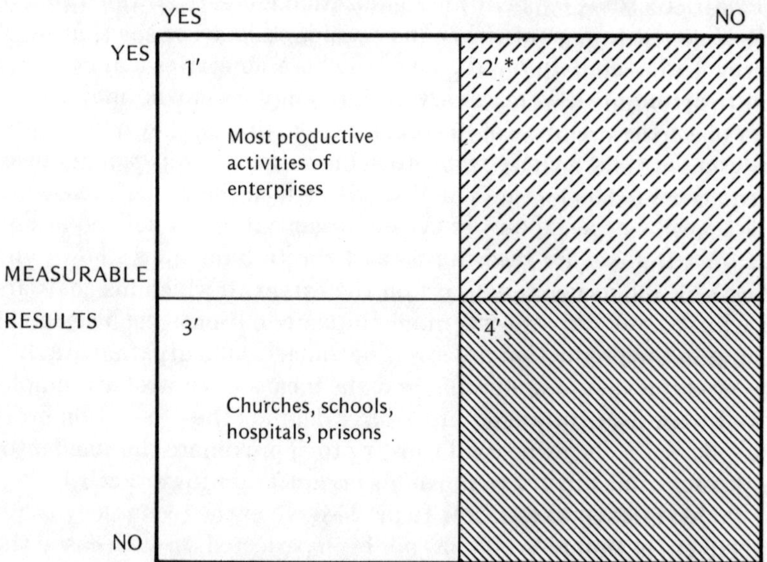

Figure 2.2. Formalized technology.

what they have, that is, salary or a position in the hierarchy. Bardach (1977), among others, has shown that people react to what they may lose—something tangible with which they are familiar—but are not sensitive to what they may gain—something that is only hypothetical. One necessary condition in overcoming their resistance would involve being able to show that the proposed change will improve the ends of the collective action. If there is no accepted way to measure these ends, it will be impossible to demonstrate the potential improvement, and the projected change will probably not take place.

Similarly, according to this principle, when an organization has two performance criteria, one measurable and the other not, the measurable criterion will be used (Riveline, 1977).

When no measurable performance criterion exists, surrogates highly influenced by culture will be substituted. Wildavsky (1977) calls this process the principle of goal displacement and maintains that "an objective that cannot be attained will be replaced by one that can be approximated." The important term implicit in Wildavsky's statement is not "approximated" but "measured" because an organization or an institution would not exist if its founders did not believe that their objectives could be attained. In spite of this fact, they are not always able to ascertain whether they have succeeded.

Change comes about differently in different organizations. In the case of organizations falling into cell 1, change may be rational and progressive: New methods can be integrated little by little because there is a consensus about what the organization should be producing, and it is possible to determine whether an alternative method is better or worse in terms of one criterion or several criteria. In organizations in cell 2 of the typology, change will be harsh and discontinuous and will come about as a consequence of the creation of another organization or institution. It will need new a priori philosophical justifications and a new paradigm that justifies the new technology. In such cases, struggles are most intense (wars of religion or conflicts among different schools in social science).

This framework can be used to analyze the health system in order to explain why certain steps to control costs and quality have been proposed and to project the efficacy of those steps.

2. MEDICAL TECHNOLOGY AND HEALTH POLICY

The consequences of medical practice in general and of hospital care in particular are not always measurable, and even when they are, there are no simple relationships between the means employed and the results obtained. When, in the interests of control, modern methods or management procedures developed for organizations in cell 1 are applied to organizations in cell 2, consequences, which will be considered below, are likely to result from the application of an inappropriate model.

Those who advocate the application of modern methods of management have been called bureaucratic rationalizers by Alford (1975). In some cases, bureaucratic rationalizers have found allies in the medical profession among the champions of scientific medicine. If medicine is a science rather than an art (Sadler, 1971; Kervasdoué and Billon, 1978), it should be possible to determine the relationship between means and ends. In the same vein, only that which can be measured is real. The body, then, is a machine that can be repaired and to which modern management methods can be applied. This perspective poses a number of problems, however, because to a large extent medical technology is cultural as well as heterogeneous. Not one but several technologies exist.

2.1. Medical Technology Is Cultural

A wealth of data supports the contention that there is not only no direct connection between medical expenditures and health but also that no link exists between inputs and outputs in the medical system. These arguments are both macro- and microeconomic.

According to the OECD (1977), per capita health expenditures in 1974 in countries having comparable life expectancies at birth varied from 750 francs per inhabitant in the United Kingdom to 2,450 francs per inhabitant in Sweden. The percentage of gross national product spent on health was 4.9 in Belgium, whereas in Sweden it was 7.4. In 1974 hospital costs accounted for less than 30 percent of health expenditures in Belgium but more than 80 percent in Sweden.

It is possible to say that there is no one method of producing medical care, that there is no production function in economic terms as there is in the automobile industry, but that there is what can be categorized a culturally-determined production function. This production function depends in fact on the history of institutions, on the compromises that have progressively characterized power struggles between the different actors in the medical system, about philosophic beliefs concerning illness and death held in a given country. All this contributes to the creation of a certain kind of health-care distribution system that lacks the rationale to be the same from country to country, especially as policies adopted in areas other than the medical sector (social laws, the power of local governments . . .) produce direct consequences on health expenditures and on the organization of the distribution of medical care. This result is quite often forgotten.

It would be possible to criticize these statements by emphasizing the fact that the link between health expenditures and life expectancy is very tenuous and that these figures cannot be matched as we purport to have done. In the words of Rudolf Klein (1977), "The activities of the NHS (British National Health Service) have very little influence on the health of the nation as a whole as measured by mortality and morbidity."

This judgment could also be made about the French, American, and German health care systems. But it is precisely because this connection is weak and because it is impossible to show the influence of health expenditure on life expectancy that such a great difference can be discerned from one country to another. To quote Rudolf Klein (1977) once again: "There are not even any agreed indicators which can be used to show whether the performance of the NHS is improving or deteriorating from one year to the next." This assertion is open to conjecture.

Passing from the macroeconomic to the microeconomic level, the phenomenon is corroborated. Jean-François Lacronique (1977) showed that the average length of hospital stay for child delivery in 1970 was 8.2 days in Finland and 13.4 days in the Netherlands, although those countries have similar perinatal and infant-mortality rates. The rate of maternal mortality is lower in Finland. The average length of stay for childbirth is as low as an average of 4.2 days in the United States, that is, three times lower than in the Netherlands.

J. F. Lacronique graphed the admission rate and the average length of stay for acute hospitalizations in a certain number of countries. (See Figure 2.3.) It is curious to note that often the countries for which the most similar figures have been recorded are those with related cultures. The admission rate and the average length of stay, therefore, have more to do with medical practice than with health, and the cost of hospitalization does not necessarily decrease because the length of stay is shorter, for admissions rates, personnel per bed, and the kind of equipment used also influence the cost.

The cost of identical treatment is very different from one country to another. According to a study made by J. R. Le Gall (1977) on the comparative cost of treating a patient in an intensive-care unit in France and the United States, the expenditure was three times less in France. This difference can be explained in part by the greater density of personnel per bed in the United States, a density that cannot, however, be explained by technical factors, for French nurses play larger medical roles than do their American counterparts.

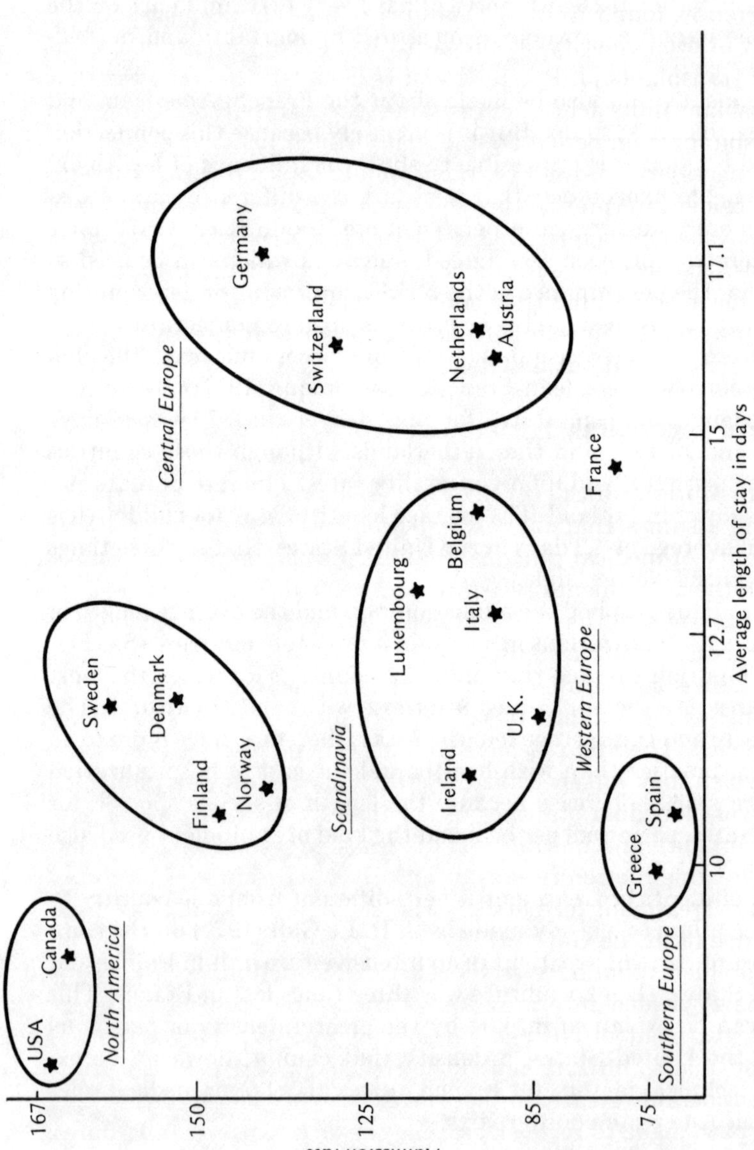

Source: J. F. Lacronique, op. cit., June 1977.

Figure 2.3. The admission rate is the number of hospital admissions per year per 1000 inhabitants.

D. Neuhauser and E. Jonsson (1974) compared coronary bypass surgery in the United States and Sweden and found that for an equivalent population, it was performed thirty-eight times more frequently in the United States than in Sweden. According to them, a certain number of factors, among which the remuneration of physicians is very important, explains this difference.

The differences found from one country to another also exist within one country or even one city. A comparative study of the cost of dialysis and kidney transplants (J. P. Grelot and H. Soufflet, 1977) showed that of two transplant units achieving the same success rate, one recorded an average hospitalization period double that of the other.

It is not necessary to dwell on these well-known data. But it seems useful to consider interpreting these figures, for two reactions may arise: The first may be characterized as "shame" and stressing the waste of public funds; the second could be based on the recognition that these differences mean something that must be understood if action is to be taken. Having said this, it is important to reiterate that medical technology is not only cultural but heterogeneous.

2.2. Medical Technology Is Heterogeneous

According to Murial Gillick (1977): "The case-by-case approach to medical planning assumes that all medical problems are subsumed under some speciality of medical practice, that all the specialities are equally proficient in the attainment of their respective ends and that there is no scarcity of resources so that all worthwhile projects can be undertaken. All of these assumptions are false."

For several reasons the allocation of material and human resources to a given branch of medical practice is not dependent on its relative therapeutic efficiency. The first reason is that doctors themselves choose the branch in which they will specialize, and their choices are determined by the prestige of individual branches rather than by their therapeutic efficiency or morbidity and mortality statistics! The second reason is that the cost of treatment often rises as its effectiveness declines. The cost of intensive-care treatment for patients who die is twice as high as for patients who live (J. R. Le Gall, 1977).

Medical problems that have as yet generated no definitive therapeutic solutions have yielded intermediate solutions that are usually very costly (the treatment of chronic kidney deficiency by dialysis; cancer radiotherapy, and so on). Although the treatment cost per year of life gained is considerably greater in these fields than in other medical areas, no call has been made to reconsider using these therapeutic procedures.

One never voluntarily chooses to let an individual die when he or she could be kept alive for months or even years in normal or nearly normal conditions. The choice is implicit, and it is forced. In any given budget there are choices to be made concerning which the application of cost/benefit studies could be useful (even though none has yielded practical results based on financial criteria alone). But in the long run the budget will rise until even marginal life-prolonging techniques are used and corresponding expenditures are incurred whatever the cost. To our knowledge, the development of medical technology has never been hindered however small (neutrontherapy, in the case of cancer) the therapeutic benefit is estimated to be. This having been said, all countries cannot offer artificial kidneys to all patients who need them. Consequently, it is considered necessary to find rationing criteria that may be medical, social, or economic. But rationing will tend to disappear because of social pressure.

The problem is different when the medical and human benefit is not obvious (Neuhauser and Jonnson, 1974). Doubt is a necessary condition governing the use of economic criteria other than budgetary constraints. When budgetary constraint exists, competition among different branches of medicine is decisive in determining the allocation of resources, and organizations and institutions play important mediating roles, as we pointed out in our study of biomedical research laboratories (J. de Kervasdoué and F. Billon, 1977).

What consequences will flow from the imposition of standards, currently being set in various West European countries, designed to control costs, improve quality, and guarantee greater equality of access to as well as a more equitable distribution of health care?

2.3. Production Norms

By production norms we mean bed/population[7] ratios as well as ratios for heavy equipment (scanners, high voltage accelerators) and personnel/bed ratios. These standards are based on two principles: the principle of equality and the principle of quality. The importance of these principles varies from one country to another.

In France the hospital law of December 31, 1970, introduced the "health-care map," the objective of which was to define "health sectors" and apply standards for equipment in each of these sectors. This law was obviously inspired by the principle of equality. Wildavsky (1977) demonstrated that:

> Every move to increase equality in one dimension necessarily decreases it in another.

Every bed/population ratio penalizes geographic areas that have low population densities. This consequence has not been ignored by the Health Ministry, which remarked in a memorandum of May 22, 1973 (DGSP/180/EC): "It is important also to take into account distances and traffic difficulties . . . without, however, allowing these factors to serve as a pretext for the survival of small institutions that do not meet equipment and care standards."

In addition to these equalitarian quantitative ratios, there are standards based on the principle of quality. It is mainly in the United States, however, that the principle of quality is important. It appears officially at the same level as the principles of equality and of cost control.

Thus in the "National Guidelines for Health Planning" presented to Congress in October 1977 by the secretary of HEW, one finds that

> obstetrics units must admit at least 2,000 deliveries a year;
> cardiac-surgery units must perform at least 200 operations a year;
> scanners must perform at least 2,500 examinations a year as the quality of scans rises with their frequency.

Furthermore, the principle of quality is nearly always in agreement with the principle of economic optimization in the use of costly equipment. Therefore, we expect the tendency to put quality before equality to result in a hospital system that is concentrated in certain urban centers rather than distributed throughout a region.

These standards suit administrators who wish to make the use of certain kinds of equipment profitable, even if "profitability" leads to overconsumption and the waste of community resources. If economic and accounting techniques sometimes prove that a specific piece of equipment is underused, they can never prove that it is overused or not used properly. This suits doctors who can not only add to the resources that they control (J. de Kervasdoué, 1973) but can also show that there is a level of use below which the technique is poorly mastered and that quality rises with increased usage. Technical motives, financial motives, and prestige lead in the same direction—away from controlling expenditure.

Maximum standards based on the equalitarian principle do not always produce the desired effects for two reasons. The first depends on the manner in which the standards have been computed and the second on the manner in which they are applied.

In France, for example, standards governing the bed capacity of the "health care map" have been defined in terms of existing equipment. The average rate of occupancy has been observed in an average region; a (slight) correcting factor has been introduced in order to take into account the expected decrease in the average length of stay. A standard ratio was produced that corresponds approximately to the national bed-equipment situation of that time (1970).

These standards allow areas that have experienced equipment ratios below the norm to expand their capacity without reducing the capacity of areas whose ratios are above the norm. In this way France, which had a total of 380,000 rate beds in 1968, made 55,000 additional beds available between 1968 and 1974. One may well wonder why beds are not eliminated. The answer is simple. It is to be found in Decree 72-352 of May 2, 1972, a "décret d'application" of the hospital law that defines the composition of the Council of Interhospital Groups whose duty is to advise on the creation and the elimination of beds and heavy equipment in private clinics in its geographic area. This council is composed primarily of doctors and hospital administrators.[8] The remaining members, usually members of hospital boards, are aware of and often defend hospital interests. It is not difficult to understand why beds are not eliminated. And even if the council were composed in a different way, it is difficult to imagine a governing body closing a hospital in a community on the grounds of applying standards, deciding why one hospital should be closed instead of another, and determining what is to be done with the employees thrown out of work. The "health-care map" also has an impact on the increasing number of specialized beds in every sector. Indicative norms produced by the Ministry of Health on bed ratios per thousand inhabitants in cardiology and other medical specialities are applicable at the sector level, not at the regional level. There are 284 sectors in France, a substantial number, leading to the situation outlined by the "Cour des Comptes" (1977): "Isolated in too narrow a district, or artificially separated by administrative boundaries from institutions with sophisticated equipment, small hospitals have a tendency to enlarge their goals: they are tempted, in particular under the impulse of their doctors, to open new medical services which would be more appropriately located in the nearest university hospital."

What is true of beds is also true of other equipment. One buys new medical equipment because the "health care map" allows such acquisitions. Again, according to the "Cour des Comptes": "In spite of the existence of such equipment [cobalt therapy unit] in a private hospital of that city, the public hospital of La Roche sur Yon wanted to have its own. It is still not used since the specialist left for Nantes. In Angoulême, public and private hospitals each have their own unit, but the former is inactive also for lack of personnel (p. 1289)."

Norm setting has led to the opposite of the intended goal by limiting the supply of medical equipment or to unintended results that are the classic consequences of limitations in supply. With respect to formal consequences, apparent conformity to existing norms can be attained in another way, simply by the artifice of combining geographic areas. The regrouping of two subzones, one underequipped and the other overequipped, can result in one zone whose equipment ratio appears to conform to the standard.

As far as rationing is concerned, the necessity of asking for a governmental authorization to create beds has led certain institutions to apply for authorizations to increase their bed capacities, which when granted, have not been followed by the construction of beds but by the resale of the authorizations to other hospitals. The same situation prevails as far as heavy equipment is concerned. For example, radiotherapy units are kept by institutions after they become obsolete and even dangerous. They are eventually resold to hospitals that wish to possess this equipment. In this way an authorization previously considered worthless acquires value. Although there is conformity with the letter of the law, its spirit is subverted, and standards of quality are not respected. A logical situation leads to absurd consequences.

These procedures are not only ineffective—after the introduction of the "health-care map," more beds became available in France than ever before—but they have also led to the classic results that flow from all systems of supply rationing. One can go further and say that even had the intended effect been attained, that is, the achievement of equivalent bed and heavy equipment to population ratios in every sector, neither geographic disparities nor expenditure would have been reduced because geographic disparities stem from varying population densities and because standardizing procedures related to expenditures are always slightly out of date. Indeed, this contention is supported by the way in which the bed/population ratio is computed: It is based on existing equipment and actual use, criteria that allow for no change in global capacity. Inasmuch as the average length of stay decreases considerably, the existing capacity is sufficient to handle hospitalization needs, even if the admission rate were to rise greatly. The norms of the map may certainly be adjusted after a slight delay, but they do not hinder supply, that is, the number of possible hospital admissions.

2.4. The Control of Quality

Paradoxically, the origin of quality control may be found in the search for cost control. The movement began on a large scale in the United States with the amendment of the Social Security Act that created the PSROs (1972).[9] This amendment was passed primarily because Congress considered it a way to stop the rapid increase in medical expenditures that failed to reflect any measurable improvement in the health of the nation. It is obvious that there is great temptation for a physician paid on a fee basis (as is the case in the United States and France) to prescribe operations, X-rays, and biological tests even in cases in which these procedures are not absolutely necessary. Numerous data exist showing that this danger is real. Thus in the "Forward Plan for Health" (1976) one reads: "In a single state, the rate of tonsillectomy varies so widely that in one hospital service area the probability that a child will have his tonsils removed is 8 percent, while in another it is 62 percent. A 1974 study of a presurgical screening program found that 24 percent of all recommended procedures were not confirmed by consultants to whom the patients were referred for a second opinion." Numerous other corroborating sources could also be quoted, but we will not dwell on this point.

In order to prevent these potential abuses, Congress wanted the practices of every physician to be examined by his or her colleagues. The law rests on two hypotheses:

1. Physicians are the most competent people to judge the quality of medical care.
2. Control must be exercised at the local level. To that end, the United States was divided into 203 regions.

Every hospitalized patient and every doctor are checked. In order to exercise this control, criteria were defined for all common pathologies, and standards were established for admission, average length of stay, and the application of therapeutic resources. The practices of each doctor in each case were examined in relation to these standards.

How will these procedures effect the cost of health care, the distribution of treatment, and health standards? The effect of these measures on health expenditure is not yet clear, but we believe that in the long term they will not stop the rise of expenditures and may even increase them. In the short and middle terms, these measures will probably result in the elimination of a certain number of questionable practices, such as unnecessary operations and a multiplicity of diagnostic procedures. But absolute proof of uselessness will have to be established before a practice is stopped, and clinical proof is not always easy to establish for methodological reasons known to doctors and social scientists. When a doubt remains, one acts according to the principle identified by Wildavsky (1977): "There is always something to do."

But once practices are brought closer to the standards desired by clinical specialists, there is no reason why this mechanism should lead to lower costs; moreover, the people in charge of the PSRO program are exercising prudence in this respect. The standards will be applied to all cases in all hospitals. It is unlikely that one standard will be set for rural hospitals and another for teaching hospitals. The principle of equality is opposed to dual standards, and such a position would be politically indefensible. The outcome will be a tendency toward the development of medical subspecialities and toward the installation of heavy equipment in the hospitals of smaller communities. Indeed, if one takes the performance of medical technique as a criterion of the health system, it should be easy to demonstrate that the subspecialists familiar with a technique will use heavy equipment more effectively. But, of course, the yardstick of efficiency is determined by subspecialists who can show that they are more efficient than their colleagues in the use of certain techniques. Doctors are evaluated by their own standards—their own ideology—the "individual" tradition in medicine (J. de Kervasdoué and F. Billon, 1977), as opposed to the "social" tradition. What counts is the doctor-patient relationship, not the health of a community. The system of quality control conceived in the United States and in the process of developing in Western Europe is not a measure of the global efficiency of the medical system and of its impact on the health of a population but a measure of the efficiency of medicine based on medical yardsticks. This system can be of interest to the patient and even to the community. To the extent that production functions obtain, medical expenditures can be planned. The consequence of this evolution would move medicine into cell 1 of our diagram, where technique and result are both defined. But not all medicine will be involved in this step, for the practice of medicine is not limited to technical roles. Despite great progress, medical technique is still at the beginning stage in many areas, where needs exist and little knowledge is available to fill them. Medicine will therefore keep part of its cultural character and, above all, its heterogeneity, which will grow with the multiplication of medical subspecialities.

2.5. Cost Control, Equality, Medical Geography, and Demography

Although problems related to the number of doctors and their geographical location could have been examined under the heading of production norms, these problems raise certain questions that justify independent analysis.

The number and the geographic distribution of physicians are indeed among the essential factors in the health policy of a nation. The number of doctors is essential because supply is the determining factor in expenditures. Geographical location is essential because it is useless to distribute medical equipment if there is no doctor to use it. This relationship usually escapes notice in the policymaking process. The number of doctors is controlled by the profession, and geographic location is usually left to personal choice that depends on the country and the availability of incentives or, conversely, on a situation in which a large number of practicing physicians results in the constraints of competition. Even in Great Britain, the most advanced country in this respect, Rudolf Klein (1977) observed that "In an open society—which respects both the direction of labour and the closing of frontiers—the ability of the State to persuade professionals to move into, say, run-down northern industrial cities or into specialities like geriatrics or mental handicap is strictly limited." In Great Britain, as anywhere else, "The reality, for the medical profession, may be State employment. The mythology, however, is still that of the self-employed practitioner." Of course, this argument is ethical: One speaks of the independence of the profession, liberty, and even medical secrecy. The result is a high density of doctors in large cities or in areas considered pleasant because of their climate or their proximity to the sea, the mountains, or a university. Thus Rogers (1977) showed that there were 50 doctors per 100,000 inhabitants in the Bronx, New York, whereas there were 239 per 100,000 inhabitants in Boston, Massachusetts, and that the gap between poor and rich areas is even greater for specialists than for general practitioners. One encounters the same phenomenon in France, where, according to the CREDOC (Research Center for the Study and Observation of Living Conditions) (H. Faure, S. Sandier, F. Tonnelier), the relative density of general practitioners varies from 1 to 2.7 according to department. This range is from 1 to 8 for specialists.[10]

How can one claim to plan medical-care production when, for ideological and political reasons, measures that would allow the attainment of the established objectives are not taken? In light of this analysis, how can the evolution of health policies in Western countries (policies having, as we have seen, many points in common) be interpreted? How can one explain the fact that despite a great wish for reform, the health system does not change? Is it possible to imagine medical techniques other than those that we already know?

Some answers to these questions can be found in Marc Renaud's (1977) article analyzing state intervention in health matters in Quebec. We shall present these answers, for they are novel, and we will indicate our points of agreement and disagreement with the author.

3. WHAT IS NEW?

The Quebec example is very interesting. The propositions made by the Castonguay-Nepveu Commission, which served as the basis for reforms made since 1970, were very ambitious. Intended to modify behavior in the health field, they were based on four broad principles:

1. Global medicine, in which the social origin of illness is recognized and the intention is to act on this knowledge as well as on somatic consequences.
2. Decentralization toward regions.
3. Participation of users and health workers in controlling organizations.
4. Equalization of rights and privileges for health workers.

These principles served as the bases for numerous reforms, laws, and administrative organizations. However, according to Renaud (1977),

> Despite the slogans which promised fundamental reform of the health sector in Quebec, in the end this reform, like that in Ontario, boiled down to a certain reallocation of resources between various elite groups. The governmental technocrats have thereby increased their powers and privileges considerably; their ideology of bureaucratic rationalization has become dominant in Quebec. Doctors made sure of the continuation of their professional domination as well as, by means of the actions of their professional organizations, a marked improvement in their working conditions. The legal status of other professionals in the health area has improved somewhat: utilization of their services has often increased and new employment opportunities have opened up. As for the population on the whole, its situation has improved in so far as health services have become free—which in itself is an extremely important "victory"—but it has obtained practically no other tangible benefit. For the population, the great ideals put forward were merely the rhetorical symbols of a changing of the guard, from doctors to governmental technocrats.

To recapitulate his explanation, during the 1960s a new middle class appeared in Quebec; it was composed of Francophones with "academic capital" who wished to be employed in their home provinces. The only possible employer was the state. This class justified the growing ascendance of the state. It was made up of "a group of technocratic elites." This group of elites was responsible for the emergence of a new ideology in the area of health, that of "bureaucratic rationalization." Those who adhered to this ideology entered into conflict with the "professional monopolizers" (doctors), but this conflict existed only on the surface. In fact, there exists a community of interests between these two groups, and their conflicts benefit them, not the population.

This is stated to be the case because "the State in a capitalist society cannot oppose the logic by which good health depends almost entirely on the production, distribution, and consumption of goods. When the State intervenes, it cannot act against the cure: consumption equation, which is the central issue of the capitalist production system and by which health problems are transformed into problems of consumption in an economic market-place." He stresses the compatibility between the capitalist organization of the economy and the "engineering" model (which we have called "technological" model) of medicine. "Global medicine" and "participation" are therefore necessarily doomed to failure.

The 1960s certainly marked the rise of the "bureaucratic rationalizer"; it is equally true that the "engineering" model is the dominant model of medicine. But are those developments characteristic of capitalist societies alone? Instead of "capitalist," should one not substitute "industrial"? Does the author take existing relationships for causes? Although the 1960s were the years in which the number of university graduates increased and health expenditure rose, can one assume that no attempt would have been made to try to reduce health expenditure even if there had been no potential unemployment among university graduates? Have the other medical paradigms proved their worth, and if so, are they acceptable to the population? Would the population consider eating less, not smoking, and abolishing individual competition in exchange for a greater life expectancy? If this were the case, would medical expenses be less? (One has to die of something.) Are there really competing paradigms? Of course, there is what is called preventive medicine, but when it is effective, it only postpones the expenditure problem. Healthy individuals will one day be ill. And the famous Chinese example often referred to in this context is not convincing: Hospital budgets are not now increasing in that country; the application of the basic rules of hygiene has produced a great leap forward in life expectancy; and the "bare-foot doctors" have contributed to social innovation. The Chinese do smoke a lot. Have they no illnesses induced by tobacco consumption? Factory safety is far from the level attained in Western countries. Have they no job-related accidents? And nothing proves that competition, "stress" endured in pursuing a successful career in the Communist party, is less intense than what we face in the West to achieve success in business, government, or politics.

It would be naïve to deny the role of the biomedical industry in health matters and not to stress certain practices that some consider harmful, particularly when they produce expenditures without real justification. But is this the only factor? Is not the identification of the capitalist state as the underlying cause a refusal to analyze more deeply? To the author technology and its cultural interpretation constrain the games played by different actors, and we do not believe that technology is entirely a product of dominant groups' interests or ideologies.

CONCLUSION

We have seen that physicians, like health-system administrators, believe in a cause-and-effect relatonship between means (resources) used and results obtained; in fact, however, medical results can only rarely be measured; and resources vary greatly from one country to another. We have demonstrated that medical practice is, on the one hand, a "cultural" phenomenon and, on the other, "heterogeneous" in nature and that consequently the use of management, planning, and control techniques does not ensure the achievement of anticipated results. We have also seen that these techniques would probably be better adapted if the movement toward controlling the quality of medical care, as it developed in the United States, were widespread but that this development would not eliminate entirely the "cultural" aspect of medicine nor would it affect the "heterogeneous" nature and effectiveness of treatment. Nor would the extension of quality control bring about a reduction in health expenditure.

We have also noted that the objective of equal access to treatment cannot be reached because there is as yet no effective way to influence physicians in choosing geographic locations for establishing their practices and that even if their choices could be influenced, equality would not exist in all dimensions.

Finally, we have examined the Canadian example and tried to analyze the failure of the reforms undertaken, showing that the strategies of the different actors described by Renaud can be interpreted with reference not to their ideology but to the state of technology that allows this ideology to exist.

This reflection could cause extreme pessimism. Such is not our purpose. Instead, it is our contention that a clear understanding of the health-care system is a necessary first step. Identifying internal contradictions and therefore the choices and trade-offs to be made will lead to the determination of appropriate techniques of management and control.

NOTES

1. Indirect evidence can be inferred from a recent survey that shows that the inhabitants of all countries of the European Economic Community place medicine at the top of the

list of priorities for scientific research. It is undeniable that the people of these nations attach great importance to this sector, for cost control implies the elimination of useless expenditures but not the limitation of expenditure when there is a potential benefit for the health of an individual, even if that impact is minimal.

2. The biological analogy, based on systems theory, has sometimes replaced the mechanical analogy. The biological one has its drawbacks also.
3. The word *technique* in French has been translated *technology* in English in order to conform to the meaning of that word used by such authors as Woodward, Thompson, Perrow, Lawrence, and Lorsch.
4. Some researchers, however, are tackling that problem.
5. "Bureaucratization" refers here to the connotations that commonly go with "bureaucracy" rather than to the sociological meaning developed by Max Weber.
6. Rules exist for other reasons and have other functions. Specifically, they protect an employee from the arbitrary power of the employer or his agent.
7. For instance, in France: 1.9 to 2.3 medical beds per thousand inhabitants, 1.9 to 2.5 surgical beds, and 0.4 to 0.5 gynecological and obstetrical beds.
8. They are twelve out of eighteen; the others are representatives of health-insurance agencies and civil servants at the departmental or the regional level.
9. At the outset, the medical profession opposed this amendment. The profession finally accepted it, however, for two reasons: (1) It is the first legal acknowledgment of the ideological position defended by the staff of major medical schools, that is, medicine is a science (as opposed to an art). (2) It is a defense against the ever-increasing number of "malpractice" suits. The medical profession as a whole is well aware of this aspect of the amendment.
10. This statement requires further comment. According to a recent study (CREDOC: H. Faure, S. Sandier, F. Tonnelier, "Regional Analysis of the Relationship between the Supply of and the Demand for Medical Care (Private Sector)," it would seem that signs are appearing that indicate the approaching saturation of the demand for the services of general practitioners; no such sign is apparent with respect to the demand for specialized medical care.

BIBLIOGRAPHY

Alford, Robert R. *Health Care Politics: Ideological and Interest Group Barriers to Reform.* Chicago and London: The University of Chicago Press, 1975.

Bardach, Eugene. *The Implementation Game: What Happens After a Bill Becomes a Law.* Cambridge, Mass.: The MIT Press, 1977.

Becker, Selwyn, and Gerald Gordon. "An Entrepreneurial Theory of Formal Organizations, Part I: Patterns of Formal Organizations." *Administrative Science Quarterly,* 11: December 1966, 315–334.

Cour des Comptes. "Rapport au Président de la République." *Journal Officiel,* 2 July 1977, 1288.

Faure, H., S. Sandier, and F. Tonnelier. "Analyse régionale des relations entre l'offre et la consommation de soins médicaux (secteur privé)" *CREDOC.*

Gillick, Muriel. "The Criteria of Choice in Medical Policy: Radiotherapy." *Massachusetts Minerva,* XV (1), Spring 1977, 15–31.

Grelot, Jean-Philippe, and Hervé Soufflet. *"L'insuffisance rénale chronique: analyse comparée de la dialyse et la transplantation."* Assistance Publique de

Paris, Centre de Recherche en Gestion, Ecole Polytechnique, January 1977.

de Kervasdoué, Jean. *"Power, Efficiency and Adoption of Innovations in Formal Organizations."* Unpublished Ph.D. Dissertation, Cornell University, 1973.

de Kervasdoué, Jean, and John Kimberly. *"Are Organizational Structures Culture Free: The Case of Hospital Innovations in the U.S. and France."* Paper presented in Honolulu, Hawaii, September 1977 to the Conference on Cross-cultural Studies on Organizational Functioning.

de Kervasdoué, Jean, and François Billon. *"Developpement de la recherche et influences externes: Le cas du cancer et des affections respiratoires."* Centre de Recherche en Gestion, Ecole Polytechnique, January 1978.

Klein, Rudolf. "The Corporate State, the Health Service and the Professions." *New University Quarterly,* 31 (2), Spring 1977.

Lacronique, Jean-François. *"Cross-sectional International Analysis of the Consumption of Short-Term Medical Care."* Unpublished Dissertation, MIT, June 1977.

Le Gall, Jean-René. Mimeo, *"Le profil du coût des soins intensifs."* Paris, 1977.

March, James, and Herbert Simon. *Organizations.* New York: Wiley, 1958.

Neuhauser, Duncan, and Edgar Jonnson. "Managerial Response to New Health Care Technology: Coronary Artery Bypass Surgery." In *The Management of Health Care,* ed. William J. Abernathy, Alan Sheldon, and Coimbatore K. Prahalad. Cambridge, Mass.: Ballinger Publishing Company, 1974.

OECD. *"Dépenses publiques de Santé,"* February 1977.

Perrow, Charles. "Hospitals: Technology, Structure and Goals." In *Handbook of Organizations,* ed. James G. March. Chicago: Rand McNally, 1965, pp. 910–931.

Renaud, Marc. "Reforme ou illusion? Une analyse des interventions de l'Etat quebecois dans le domaine de la santé." *Sociologie et Sociétés,* 9 (1), April 1977.

Riveline, C. "Esquisse d'une nouvelle économie d'entreprise." *Annales des Mines,* April 1977.

Rogers, David E. "The challenge of primary care." *Daedalus,* Winter 1977, 81–103.

Sadler, Judith. *"Ideologies of 'Art' and 'Science' in Medicine: The Transition from Medical Care to the Application of Technique in the British Medical Profession."* Memo, University of Manchester, 1977.

Stephan, Jean-Claude. *"Economie et Pouvoir Médical."* Economica édit., Paris, 1978.

Thomas, Lewis. "On the Science and Technology of Medicine." *Daedalus,* Winter 1977, 35–46.

U.S. Department of Health, Education and Welfare, *Public Health Service. Forward Plan for Health.* FY 1978–1982. *August 1976, p. 60.*

Wildavsky, Aaron. "Doing better and feeling worse." *Daedalus,* Winter 1977, 105–123.

Chapter 3

Innovation and the Health Services Sector: Notes on the United States

T. R. Marmor and James A. Morone

It is difficult to exaggerate the changes that have characterized the discussion of American medicine over the past decade. Some of these changes are common across the developed economies, but some do not particularly affect innovation. Nonetheless, before addressing the topic of innovation in health-delivery arrangements, some attention should be given to the context in which innovation has developed.

INTRODUCTION

Over the last decade the economic and moral problems of medicine, as Paul Starr recently characterized the dilemna,[1] have displaced scientific progress at the center of public attention. The presumption about the future is that costs will increase; the presumption about corresponding improvements in health is that they are doubtful. Precisely how different a perception of the world these presumptions reflect can be discerned by contrasting them with the prevailing beliefs of the early 1960s.

The premise of social policy then was that the United States needed and would benefit from more medical care. Federal programs were directed toward increasing resources in the field and augmenting the financial resources of the old and the poor so that they could purchase care. There was a program for each problem, but considerable slippage occurred between the program launched and the problem to be solved.[2] More legislation, more resources, and better government—this phrase was the trinity that President Johnson invoked when he proudly asserted that during his administration "40 national health measures were presented to the Congress and passed by the Congress—more than in all the preceding 175 years of the Republic's history." [3]

Precisely how much the assumptions have changed is suggested by the old-fashioned quality of Johnson's satisfaction. In none of the OECD countries today is more medical care the central preoccupation. If there is any central concern, it is how to get less or, at the very least, how to reduce the rate of increase in medical-care claims that must be met by public expenditures. Those who shape policy express the reversal of assumptions underlying the programs that they laud or the innovations that they sponsor. It is by no means an accident that even beyond the Canadian border, the most widely-read document on Canadian health policy was not about health insurance but about "new perspectives on the health of Canadians." [4] These new perspectives stressed the limits of medicine's impact on health, the opportunities that individuals have to improve their own health, and the collective efforts—in pollution control, accident prevention, and tax policy regarding food and drink—still open to the Canadian government.

The issues of debate, of course, are not the same across Europe and North America. But the preoccupation with controlling costs and the loss of faith in a technologically-innovative and improving medical-care system is widespread. As a result, even a discussion of the title of this volume—Innovation in Health Policy and Service Delivery—is likely to be shaped by the current orthodoxy regarding the problems of medicine.

INNOVATION IN HEALTH SERVICES DELIVERY

The major contention that we make is quite simple. The medical-care industry *is* characterized by very high levels of innovation: in technology, in drugs and treatment, and in the site and in the arrangement of care. The care delivered is subject to frequent change (witness cancer therapies). The instruments employed in diagnosis and treatment have short lives. And even the places where physicians work—whether in offices outside hospitals or inside, alone or in groups—have altered dramatically in the last quarter century, at least in North America. In contrast to law or teaching, medicine is an innovative profession; its professionals are used to changes in their work, their interventions, their rules, and their facilities that are, by comparative professional standards, quite striking.

That claim, of course, will not go unchallenged. In order to focus the discussion, it may be helpful to explain precisely what one means when one maintains that the profession is hostile to innovation in delivery arrangements. What is meant is simply that medical professionals resist both cost containment and restraints on professional autonomy. The problem does not involve resistance to change in general but to particular kinds of changes. Some professions—and teaching comes to mind—are more resistant to changes in general. The differences will become clear by contrasting two major items of medical care innovation: changes in technology that are welcomed by the profession, as opposed to changes in financing and the delivery of services that are resisted by the profession.

MEDICAL TECHNOLOGY AND INNOVATION

Technological change has dominated our understanding of medicine's recent past. The so-called CAT scanner is only the most recent in a long series of dramatic technological developments in medicine. New techniques for heart surgery, means for transplanting tissues and organs, and—to recall previous decades—a long series of innovations in drug research testify to a belief in inevitable medical progress through technological innovation.

In recent years this faith has been questioned. Various programs have been devised to control the "overuse" of new technologies; we call them PSROs, or Professional Standards Review Organizations. Apart from overuse, the regulations increasingly reflect questions concerning whether technological improvements are worth the cost.

And the cost—particularly the cost for use and maintenance, as opposed to purchase—can be substantial. CAT scanners, for instance, currently range in price from $250,000 to $650,000. Operating costs add $300,000 to $500,000 a year, and professional fees for performing the scans add still another $200,000. As a paradigmatic example of the costs of technical medical progress, CAT scanners reveal the clash between cost containment and technical innovation.[5]

The example of the CAT scanner is now commonly employed to show how technology and formal medical care have been overly stressed in the pursuit of health objectives. And there is no doubt about the increased consciousness of personal health habits and environmental conditions. Joggers, health-food stores, and the increased popularity of racquet games attest to the new consciousness about health habits. How faddish and transient this development may be cannot yet be determined; but it does signal some awareness of the limits of medicine, which would have seemed unorthodox even a decade ago.

On an environmental level, numerous groups have tried to redress the imbalance of political markets. Their impact is uneven, but it is not negligible. Cigarette advertisements no longer finance television programs, even though federal subsidies to tobacco farmers continue. Auto emission standards have been mandated, although compliance has been delayed. Standards for reduced water pollution have been set, although enforcement has generated controversy everywhere.

Paralleling changes in attitudes toward personal and environmental health questions is the backlash against technologically-sophisticated medical research and care practices. Asserting that in this arena "less is better," reformers like Carlson, Ardell, and others have challenged high-technology medicine and demanded alternative settings for care and more emphasis on humaneness rather than on the scientific credentials of those who provide care.[6] Some would point to the interest in "natural" childbirth as an illustration; the advocacy of home birth as an alternative and midwives as substitutes for obstetricians expresses this cast of mind. At the most extreme, there is a virulent distrust of institutional medicine, exemplified by Ivan Illich's contention that most disease in America is iatrogenic, that is, caused by the health system itself. It may well be that the dismissal of clinical medical care is the obverse example of the myopia that formerly overlooked life styles and the environment as factors in illness. Nonetheless, this kind of skepticism marks a significant break with earlier affirmations of faith in the inevitable progress of scientific medical care.

The political implications of this skepticism are difficult to predict. They may be indirect. For example, efforts to control costs may gain in legitimacy with the spread of doubt about the efficacy of medical care. What was considered best about American medicine—the application of its research and high technology—may in some areas be reversed, supporting a demand for restricting the application of research and medical technology. On the one hand, the discussion of medicine may be changed permanently by the new advocates; on the other, these bursts of opinion are vocal rather than widespread and will not in the short term effect the radical transformation of the system of delivering care. For insight into that possible transformation, one must turn to the critics who regard medical care as valuable but consider its organization, delivery, and financing arrangements perverse.

THE MOVEMENT FOR HEALTH MAINTENANCE ORGANIZATIONS

The most concerted and widely advertised movement for change in the delivery of medical care has focused for almost a decade on health maintenance organizations, or what the last generation called prepaid group practices or community-health centers. HMOs, as their promoters state, are "organizations which provide comprehensive health services to voluntarily enrolled consumers on the basis of fixed price or capitation contracts."[7] Because consumers prepay a fixed annual amount, providers of care have financial incentives to economize on costs. Ideally, providers substitute adequate but less-costly treatment for more-costly care, curb excessive use, and emphasize preventive medicine. Voluntary enrollment (and disenrollment), it is hoped, prevents the underprovision of care.

HMOs constitute an appealing innovation because they address directly the way in which fee-for-service reimbursement contributes to medical-care inflation. Reimbursing providers for services rendered rewards the rendering of more services. And with the spread of insurance, the most direct patient pressure against the casual use of medical-care resources has been reduced. HMOs not only turn away from fee reimbursement but also address the problems of service fragmentation by organizing a full range of services under one roof. This at least was the case made for them.

In 1971 President Nixon placed HMO development at the center of his program to reduce the rate of medical-care inflation. The Nixon administration seemed to confront the traditional preference of American physicians for fee reimbursement. But in practice, the Nixon plan expanded to include fee-for-service groups; in effect this expansion undermined one of HMO's major features that involved building a coalition of support. Abandoning exclusive capitation was merely one element in an inflated rhetorical campaign. There was "something for everyone" in this systemic panacea; the reality could not fail to cause disappointment.[8]

One should note the similarity of HMOs to the neighborhood health centers of the Johnson period. Both were touted as major innovations in the organization and delivery of care. Both were intended to overcome problems of access, fragmentation, and funding. The neighborhood centers, however, had mostly poor, disorganized clienteles for support and experienced slow growth and eventual funding reversals. HMOs, by contrast, were promoted in a form that promised "something for everyone." The 1973 act, although unsuccessful in promoting the significant growth of HMOs, is still considered the expression of a viable policy option today.[9]

The fate of the Nixon administration's major innovation is instructive. Standards for federal subsidies were set so high that not only new HMOs but existing, successful ones (the models for the law) failed to meet the criteria for funds. Few even applied. Between 1974 and 1977, only 70 million dollars were disbursed, although 250 million had been authorized. And the HMOs that did grow produced a set of scandalous side effects for the poor in the Medicaid program that linger to this day.

Although general-purpose HMOs grew slowly, there was a burst of activity in ones directed at the Medicaid population, and expectations were inflated. The poor, it was claimed, would get mainstream medicine at low cost. In California 55 HMOs signed up 237,000 Medicaid recipients in 1974; 58 of the 77 California HMOs had Medicaid contracts. The aftermath was a disaster. A series of sensational investigations documented marketing fraud, the underprovision of services, poor treatment, and, as it turned out, exorbitant administrative costs (approximately 50 percent of program expenditures). Tighter controls, which most HMOs would or could not meet, were imposed. By 1977 the number of Medicaid HMOs in California had dropped from 58 to 18, providing care to 150,000 persons. No longer is there any pretense that such organizations provide their patients with mainstream medicine.[10]

For reasons too complicated to detail here, there are substantial barriers to HMO growth in federal policy itself. The problems arise from the tax code, the rules of Medicare, and the complications of the HMO act. Still HEW continues to adjust the regulations, and proposals for growth continue to be formulated. The inflated expectations with which HMOs were originally launched continue to plague this innovation. It is, as one commentator noted, one alternative, not *the* alternative system for delivering and financing care.

A CONCLUDING REMARK

The issue of innovation in the delivery of medical care is not a simple one. The question is not whether powerful groups in medical care will accept innovation. They have. They will accept changes in the site, content, and technological complements of medical services that promise improved care without threats to professional prerogatives. In this brief comment, the case of CAT scanners has been used to illustrate the technological innovation that marks American medicine. By contrast, the exaggerated hope for innovations in the financing of medical care—particularly HMOs—illustrates the barriers to innovation that threaten the traditional preferences of physicians. Considerably less than one-tenth of American health expenditures now occur in HMO settings. Discussions of innovation that emphasize this or any other instrument to the exclusion of others are likely to overlook innovations that will affect the health care delivered to most citizens in the United States or in any other advanced industrial nation.

There is a connection between the two topics of this essay that should be iterated at its conclusion. The acceptance of innovative technology related to hospital medicine and biomedical research has contributed to the political controversy over medical-care costs that, for example, the group-practice model has addressed. Whereas some propose great organizational modes of financing and organizing medical practice as a panacea for medical-care inflation, that is not the position adopted here. On the contrary, what will be required, in our view, are innovative modes of negotiation and bargaining over the direction of investment in medical care. As faith in medical progress through scientific innovation wanes, the search for ways to balance claims in this sector will become more important. In this respect, the formulation of innovations such as HMOs represents a search for a less conflictual solution than bargaining about allocations in a sector where the growth rates of the past decade cannot be maintained amid constrained national and individual budgets.

NOTES

1. Paul Starr, "Medicine and the Waning of Professional Sovereignty," paper prepared for the Daedalus Conference, January 28–29, 1977, Washington, D.C., 1977, pp. 2–3.
2. Andrew B. Dunham and Theodore R. Marmor, "Federal Policy and Health: Recent Trends and Different Perspectives," in Theodore J. Lowi and Alan Stone (eds.), *Nationalizing Government: Public Policies in America* (Beverly Hills–London: Sage Publications, 1978), pp. 263–298.
3. Lyndon B. Johnson, *The Vantage Point: Perspectives on the Presidency,* 1963–1969 (New York: Holt, Rinehart and Winston, Inc.), 1971, p. 220.
4. Claim by one of the authors of the Lalonde Report, H. F. Lafambroise, in an interview in Chicago, April 16, 1978.
5. See Institute of Medicine, *A Policy Statement: Computer Tomographic Scanning* (Washington, D.C.: National Academy of Sciences, April 1977).
6. See, for example, Rick Carlson, *The End of Medicine* (New York: John Wiley & Sons, 1975).
7. Paul Ellwood, "Restructuring the Health Delivery System," in *Health Maintenance Organizations: A Reconfiguration of the Health Services System.* Proceedings of the Thirteenth Annual Symposium on Hospital Affairs. University of Chicago, Chicago, Illinois, May 1971, p. 4.
8. Bruce Spitz, "Medicaid Cost Containment Policy: HMO Regulation and Reimbursement" (Washington, D.C.: The Urban Institute, April 1977), working paper, p. 12.

9. See, for example, Alain Enthoven's proposed NHI plan and its central role for HMOs, submitted to HEW Secretary Califano in September 1977. "Consumer Choice Health Plan: An Approach to National Health Insurance Based on Regulated Competition in the Private Sector."
10. Bruce Spitz, *op cit.*, p. 25ff.

Chapter 4

Regulation of Capital Investments of Hospitals in the United States: Certificate-of-Need Controls

Thomas W. Bice

INTRODUCTION

Those of you who are familiar with the history of relationships between government and economic enterprises in the United States may find the topic of regulation out of place in a volume devoted to *innovations* in public services. In its various forms government regulation of private business has existed since the beginning of our Republic. The creation in 1797 of government-owned and operated hospitals for the merchant marine marked our first experience with what some call pejoratively "socialized medicine." Although government regulation of the health-services industry is not new in a historical sense, the particular forms of controls developed for and applied to the health-care industry are innovative. Therefore we have only the most meager evidence on which to base a prediction about what their effects will be on the performance of our health-services industry and seemingly only the slightest concern about their implications for traditional federal-state relationships. In view of the significance of the trend toward government management of the health-care industry via regulation and the recent and rapid extension of its application, the subject may appropriately be considered an "innovation in public services."

Because regulation is a category of government activity that subsumes several functions and mechanisms, each devised in order to attain a variety of socially desirable ends, this chapter deals with only one instance, namely, that of *regulating health-care institutions' capital-investment behavior by means of certificate-of-need (CON) controls.* The chapter specifically describes the origins, purposes, and structure of those controls and presents findings from a nationwide study of their impact on hospital-investment behavior and per capita health-care costs. As an introduction to these subjects, we define a few terms and sketch the background of the political economy of the health-care industry in the United States that has created and sustained the apparent need for government regulation. After describing the study of CON controls done by David S. Salkever (of the Johns Hopkins University) and the author,[1] we speculate about current and future policy issues regarding national health insurance and their implications for government regulation.

REGULATION

In general, regulation is a form of control aimed at creating and maintaining equilibrium. As a government activity applied to the economy or some segment of it, regulation is intended to promote and preserve the general welfare by proscribing particular economic behavior that is considered to be inimical to that end or by prescribing or encouraging other behavior that is deemed to be in the public interest. Government regulation can thus be distinguished from government ownership of the means of producing goods and services and from the government's roles as a buyer and a seller of goods and services in competitive markets. Regulation implies *indirect* control over the economic behavior of private persons by means of administrative mechanisms that are mandated statutorily and implemented by public persons.[2]

The variety of public persons and the kinds of administrative mechanisms involved in the regulatory structure of the United States are too numerous and complex to describe here. But it should be stated that regulatory controls have been applied historically in the United States by three principal kinds of agencies: (1) regulatory commissions created statutorily by legislatures and appointed by executives, (2) agencies of the executive branches of the federal and state governments, and, (3) more recently, private persons to whom the government has delegated authority to control the behavior of other private persons. All three kinds of regulators are involved in controlling segments of the health-care industry. However, one of the intriguing features of regulation in the health-services industry is its reliance on the third kind, that is, the delegation of authority to private persons. Under the banner of "voluntarism" in health-services planning, various "quasi public" bodies have recently been created to advise government agencies and (in some instances) to decide matters pertaining to the application of regulatory controls. These delegations and arrangements have given rise to peculiarities in the political economy of health-services regulation. Their implications for CON controls are discussed in the following section.

The four general kinds of regulatory mechanisms that correspond roughly to their objectives are listed below.[3]

1. Subsidies
2. Entry restrictions
3. Rate (or price) controls
4. "Quality" controls.

Subsidies are transfers of cash or other resources from the government to private persons. When provided to buyers, they are intended to stimulate demand for goods and services that are considered socially desirable and underconsumed by at least some segments of society. Subsidies to suppliers are designed to encourage production of socially-desirable goods and services. In both cases, government intervention is predicated on the belief that the market is an inefficient means of supplying and allocating particular goods and services that are deemed to enhance the general welfare.

Entry restrictions, as the term implies, govern access to the privilege of producing certain goods and services. In some instances, the government controls entry into markets in order to allocate scarce resources (for example, franchising air waves) or to promote economic efficiency by preventing ruinous competition among several suppliers when a smaller number of suppliers is deemed better (for example, natural monopolies). In other instances, which are more traditionally invoked in the health-service industry, entry restrictions are applied to promote quality and ensure the safety of buyers. Potential suppliers are allowed to enter markets only after fulfilling requirements that are intended to demonstrate their competence to produce effective and safe goods and services (for example, professional licensing).

Rate (or price) controls are imposed to limit rates (or prices) charged by suppliers of goods and services. Frequently these controls are applied along with entry restrictions as a quid pro quo that suppliers accept in return for the privilege of noncompetition that entry restrictions create. (The combination of entry restrictions and rate [or price] controls is known as public-utility regulation.)

Finally, "quality" controls are comprised of a variety of mechanisms and objectives. In general, they are aimed at assuring buyers of the efficacy and safety of goods and services (for example, the Federal Drug Administration and the Consumer Products Safety Commission) or at establishing and maintaining safe and salubrious environments, whether within settings where goods and services are produced or more generally within the larger environment. "Quality" controls differ from entry restrictions aimed at ensuring efficacy and safety inasmuch as "quality" controls are applied to suppliers periodically *after* their entry into markets.

Figure 4.1 illustrates these kinds of regulatory mechanisms, showing examples of particular instances from the health-services industry. As the columns indicate, several kinds apply to individuals—both buyers and suppliers in the case of subsidies—and others deal with corporate persons. In general, subsidies to individuals and to corporate persons and entry restrictions applied to individuals were instituted relatively early in our history. Entry restrictions imposed on corporate persons were instituted only within the past fifteen years; the regulation of rates (or prices) and "quality" controls are now being developed.[4]

Regulatory Mechanisms \ *Objects of Regulation*	Individuals	Organizations
Subsidies	Medicare Medicaid Tax credits for private insurance	Construction subsidies Grants to medical schools for medical education Loans, loan guarantees ⋮
Entry Restrictions	Licensing of professionals	Investment controls (e.g., CON)* Licensing
Rate or Price Controls	Control of MDs' fees (e.g., ESP)*	Hospital rate setting
"Quality" Controls	Peer review (e.g., PSRO)*	Accreditation (e.g., JCAH)*

* CON: Certificate of Need
ESP: Economic Stabilization Program
PSRO: Professional Standard Review Organization
JCAH: Joint Commission on the Accreditation of Hospitals

Figure 4.1. Kinds of regulation.

THE POLITICAL ECONOMY OF THE HEALTH-SERVICES INDUSTRY

A remarkable result of the rapid and extensive diffusion of regulatory programs applied exclusively to the health-care industry is that particular efforts are frequently aimed at remedying problems created by others. A widely-cited argument holds that the imposition of entry restrictions and rate controls on health-care institutions and "quality" controls on physicians is necessary because of the "failure of the market" to establish supply/demand equilibria with respect to quantities and kinds of services provided and to allocate them equitably. Others note that these presumed "market failures" originated to a great extent in earlier regulatory interventions, particularly the pricing effects of subsidized insurance and the combined supply and pricing effects stemming from subsidies and entry restrictions applied to suppliers.

Subsidies and entry restrictions, coupled with medical practice acts (adopted at the insistence of physicians), that have historically disallowed the "corporate practice of medicine" have created an industry riddled with perverse incentives. "Deep" insurance coverage leads buyers to overconsume insured health services (or at least to consume services that they might value differently were they to pay the full cost of producing them at the time of purchase). Supply subsidies and cost-based reimbursement by insurers (government and private) fuel the industry's expansion into high-cost markets, often in the name of "quality enhancement." This tendency is reinforced by the peculiar relationship of physicians to hospitals. Physicians are users and sometimes masters of hospital facilities and personnel but have only minor responsibilities for their efficient management. However, physicians have de facto control over the destinies of hospitals by virtue of their freedom to boycott the use of particular institutions. Because hospitals need patients (especially high-cost, insured patients) to maintain their cash flows and their existence, physicians exercise tremendous power over decisions about the quantity and the quality of equipment, personnel, and services that particular hospitals supply.

These fiscal and structural features of the health-care industry combine with technological change and the enduring belief on the part of the public that the close relationship between medical care and medical cure and health produces the cost-inflation problem that the United States shares with other industrialized nations. In consequence, these nations are developing sets of solutions that rest heavily on the hope that regulatory controls will deter cost inflation and preserve high-quality health services for all who need them.

One such effort in the United States employs varieties of entry restrictions on health-care institutions by attempting to control their capital investment behavior. Prominent among these restrictions are certificate-of-need (CON) laws, which, in accordance with the National Health Planning and Resources Development Act of 1974 (P.L. 93-641), are slated for adoption by all the states in the United States. As of 1972, about half of our states had adopted and implemented some version of CON. The study described in the following section attempted to evaluate their impact on hospital-investment behavior and hospital costs (more accurately, on expenditures for hospital services).

CERTIFICATE-OF-NEED CONTROLS

Background

The purpose of investment controls is to moderate cost inflation by limiting the capital investments of health-care institutions to those that are administratively certified as needed by their communities. The rationale for this approach is based principally on two arguments: One points to the substitution of inpatient for outpatient services, the other to the effects of "overcapacity" on cost inflation. The former argument notes that the use of inpatient services is associated with their supply. As hospital beds are added, their use increases. On the assumption that much of the care rendered in hospital settings could be provided as effectively in other, low-cost settings, proponents of investment controls argue that tighter supplies of inpatient facilities will force the substitution of other treatment modalities and thereby lower total health-care expenditures without compromising the quality of care. The "overcapacity" argument points to the inflationary effects of empty hospital beds and idle equipment and facilities. Because unused capacity entails the payment of fixed costs, its elimination via investment controls will also moderate total expenditures.

The case for investment controls has appealed to policymakers in the United States. Beginning with New York in the mid-1960s and continuing to the present, states have enacted CON laws. By 1972 about half had done so. In that year the federal government adopted the Section 1122 Amendment to the Social Security Act, which provides funds for states to implement investment controls similar to CON programs,[5] and in 1974 the National Health Planning and Resources Development Act (P.L. 93-641) made eligibility for the receipt of several kinds of federal subsidies contingent on the implementation of CON programs by the states.

Before 1974, the administrative structures through which CON controls were implemented and the provisions of the laws differed among the states. Most, however, relied on areawide, voluntary health-planning agencies comprised of health professionals and consumers to perform initial reviews of investment proposals and to make advisory recommendations to an agency of the state government that decided whether to issue or deny requests. This general approach is employed under the current national health-planning program.

The particular kinds of facilities covered by the laws and the kinds of sanctions levied varied among the states, but virtually all states regulated investments of hospitals, and most reviewed nursing homes as well. Under P.L. 93-641, states must review the investment plans of hospitals, nursing homes, and other specified health-care institutions.

The Study

In 1974 David S. Salkever and the author began a study of the impact of CON programs on hospital investment patterns and expenditures for hospital services. The study focused on the period from 1968 to 1972, using states as the unit of analysis. This period was chosen to minimize the potential contaminating effects of the several and varied kinds of regulatory programs that appeared after 1972.

We first examined the effects of CON controls on three investment variables, namely, (1) overall investment (measured by changes in total plant assets), (2) investment in increased capacity (measured by changes in numbers of hospital beds), and (3) investment in improvements in the quality or capital intensiveness of services (measured by changes in plant assets per bed). As shown in Figure 4.2, we expected these variables—each measuring an aspect of investment decisions—to be influenced by several exogenous factors and CON controls (Arrow A).

In the second stage of our analysis we employed the quantitative estimates of the effects of CON controls on investment decisions to estimate the impact of regulation on price-output decisions (measured by hospital per diem charges and use) and, finally, per capita expenditures for hospital services (respectively, Arrows C and D).

Findings

Our analyses indicated that CON controls did not moderate hospital-cost inflation during the 1968–1972 period. Indeed, they suggested that the programs in effect at that time might have caused slight increases in per capita expenditures for hospital services. This result was caused by

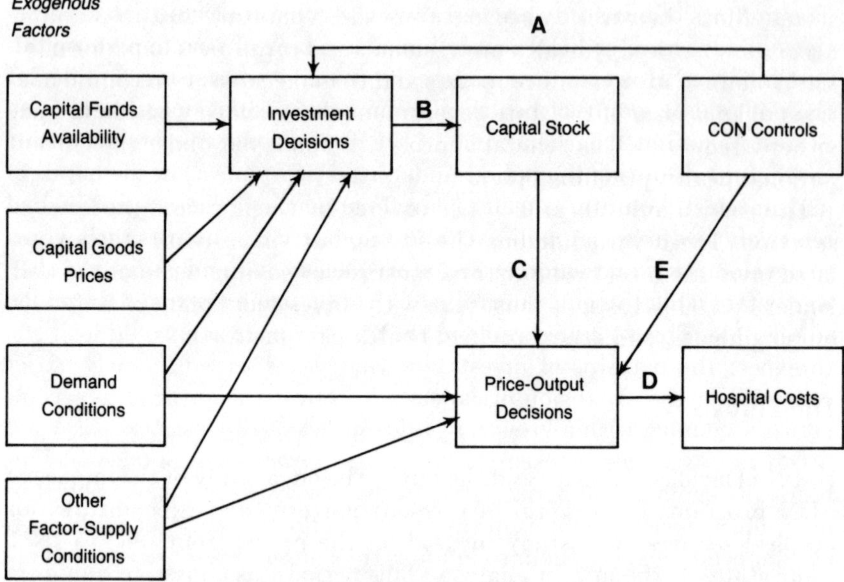

Figure 4.2. Conceptual framework for hospital cost determination.

several intervening effects. CON regulation had no detectable impact on overall investment. Given changes in the various exogenous factors that influence investment decisions (which were statistically adjusted), average total investment among states with CON programs was similar to that among states with no investment controls. However, we found clear evidence of the effects of CON programs on the *kinds* of investments made. Specifically, CON regulation *slowed* the expansion of capacity and *encouraged* the growth of investment in capital-intensive services.

This pattern of investment produced competing cost implications. On the one hand, the slower expansion of capacity in states with investment controls was accompanied by lesser increases in hospital admissions and total patient days, which slowed increases in per capita expenditures. On the other hand, the increased investment in capital-intensive services in the regulated states resulted in higher average per diem charges, thus tending to increase per capita expenditures. These competing influences were approximately offsetting, resulting in either a negligible or a slightly positive net effect on average per capita expenditures for hospital services in 1972.

Interpretation

The findings of our study are certainly not consistent with the expectations of advocates of CON regulation as a means of stemming hospital-cost inflation. However, neither are they entirely surprising considering the political economy of health planning and regulation in the United States. As we noted earlier, much of the responsibility for implementing CON controls during the period under investigation was in the hands of multiinterest, voluntary health-planning agencies. These agencies had relatively few financial, political, and information resources with which to develop plans and enforce regulatory decisions. In consequence, they were vulnerable to being controlled by those whom they were intended to regulate. This so-called capture theory[6] of regulation would lead one to expect the patterns of investment that we observed, namely, strict control over the expansion of capacity and over the entry of new competitors, coupled with a growth in price-increasing investment.

Our results are also consistent with a less extreme view of relationships between regulators and regulated firms. Given the need of voluntary planning agencies to maintain the image of effective and fair public bodies, one would expect them to employ their limited resources to pursue visible successes and avoid obvious failures.[7] In the context of health-care planning and regulation, these incentives would lead an agency to exercise strict control over the expansion of capacity and be more lax with respect to "quality-enhancing" services. The opposite strategy, which would permit the building of hospitals and the creation of beds in existing ones, could result in visible indications of failure, namely, empty hospital beds. By contrast, the effects of an overly strict control of bed growth would be less visible, for longer waiting time attends admissions for nonemergency services.

Agencies face a different set of potential rewards and sanctions when reviewing proposals for investment in new services and equipment. Tight control over these kinds of investment opens the agency to the criticism leveled by the public and the medical profession of denying citizens access to the "latest and best" medical technology. However, permitting only a few hospitals in a community to upgrade their services may be viewed as favoritism by the hospitals and medical staffs who are denied the opportunity to improve their services. Because low productivity associated with the excess capacity of particular services and pieces of equipment is not highly visible, the pressures on agencies to approve requests that do not involve the construction of beds are likely to prevail.

The tendencies to deny requests for new beds while being more permissive with respect to new services and equipment are probably reinforced by the compositions, processes, and authorities of agencies charged with implementing CON and by the vagueness of the statutes that create these programs. As we noted in the opening section of this paper, regulatory programs in the health-services industry involve private corporations, usually in de jure advisory capacities to government agencies charged ultimately with rendering regulatory decisions. Such corporations participating in health-services planning and regulation are required by statute to be constituted from various interest groups, including consumers and providers of health services. Because the language of statutes creating these programs and agencies, as well as their interrelationships with government, is typically vague with respect to functions and global with respect to purposes, much latitude remains for various actors to fill in details in ways that can be self-serving. In consequence, local advisory agencies and government officials often disagree about the authority that each commands, and local interest groups that rarely pay the full costs of investments are inclined to want more and "better" services than those who, from their perspectives at the pinnacle of the cost-inflation problem, see their total cost implications. Hence local agencies are inclined to use CON to improve the "quality" and the availability of services, whereas government agencies (particularly those responsible for health-service budgets) are apt to employ those controls to contain costs. The continued rise in costs has led government officials imbued with faith in regulation to support more vigorously the imposition of rate regulation along with "tighter" investment controls.

IMPLICATIONS

The principal lesson to be drawn from our study is that investment controls are weak deterrents of hospital-cost inflation. In our view, this results from strong pressures exerted on hospitals to improve the quality of their services and from the relatively meager financial and political resources that regulatory agencies can draw on to combat those pressures. In this connection two broad policy strategies have recently been proposed in the United States: a regulatory strategy and a market-oriented approach.

The regulatory strategy assumes that "market failures" are so pervasive within the health-services industry that more stringent and extensive regulation is required in order to reverse the trend. Since 1972 several states that were among the first to adopt CON controls have pursued this logic in adopting various forms of rate-setting programs to regulate hospitals' prices and budgets, and a few are considering proposals to impose ceilings on allowable capital expenditures. Moreover, the cost-containment strategy proposed by the Carter administration (and rejected by Congress) would have established nationwide rate-setting and investment ceilings in conjunction with investment controls.

The market-oriented approach assumes that several of the presumed "market failures" within the health-services industry can be attributed to various forms of government intervention and that their proscription would obviate the need for investment controls and other kinds of regulation currently under consideration. Advocates of this approach favor providing individuals with a greater range of options in insurance coverage, coinsurance, and deductibles and encouraging the growth of prepaid health-care plans that would place a larger portion of the risk for hospital costs on physicians.

The current stalemate in the debate about national health insurance in the United States stems from uncertainty regarding which of these policy alternatives or combinations should be pursued. Policymakers have learned from experience with Medicare and Medicaid that infusing additional money into the health-services industry as it is now structured will only exacerbate inflationary tendencies. Recent studies of particular regulatory programs, such as that described in this paper, indicate that existing approaches have produced a limited impact on cost inflation. Furthermore, it is becoming clear that strong political and economic interests resist both the more extensive regulatory strategies and the market-oriented approaches. Under these circumstances, it is doubtful that an all-encompassing national health insurance scheme with universal entitlement will be forthcoming in the United States in the foreseeable future.

NOTES

1. D. S. Salkever and T. W. Bice, "The Impact of Certificate-of-Need Controls on Hospital Investment," *Milbank Memorial Fund Quarterly/Health and Society* (Spring 1976), 185–214; "Certificate-of-Need Legislation and Hospital Costs," in M. Zubkoff, I. E. Raskin, and R. S. Hanft (eds.), *Hospital Cost Containment: Selected Notes for Future Policy* (New York: Prodist, 1978), 429–460.
2. The word *persons* is employed in the general legal sense to refer to individuals (natural persons) and organizations (corporate persons).
3. G. J. Stigler, "The Theory of Economic Regulation," *Bell Journal of Economics and Management Science,* 2 (Spring 1971), 3–21.
4. For descriptions of several of these programs and summaries of the rather limited findings presented in studies of their impact, see Zubkoff, Raskin, and Hanft, *op. cit.* For instances of critiques, see C. C. Havighurst, "Controlling Health Care Costs: Strengthening the Private Sector's Hand," *Health Politics, Policy, and Law,* 1 (Winter 1977), 471–498, and D. S. Salkever, "Will Regulation Control Health Care Costs," *Bulletin of the New York Academy of Medicine,* 54 (January 1978), 73–83.

5. The principal difference between these programs and CON laws is the kind of sanction employed. Under 1122, financial sanctions are applied whereby hospitals that engage in capital projects without prior certification lose eligibility for payment of associated costs under Medicare and Medicaid. CON laws typically impose legal sanctions, such as the revocation of licenses and fines.
6. G. Hilton, "The Basic Behavior of Regulatory Commissions," *American Economic Review* (May 1972), 47–54.
7. R. G. Noll, "The Consequences of Public Utility Regulation of Hospitals," in Institute of Medicine, *Controls on Health Care* (Washington, D.C.: National Academy of Sciences, 1975), 25–48.

PART II

Medical Technology: Public Policy and Trade-offs in Costs, Diagnosis, and Impersonal Care

With reference to developments in European and North American countries, David Banta reviews recent responses, mainly of American policymakers, to what appears to be an increasing dilemma in most industrial nations. Once praised as the benefactor of mankind and the symbol of medical and social progress, expensive high-technology medicine is increasingly being questioned in terms of its positive *and* negative consequences, its risks and prospects, as well as its economic and social costs not only to individuals but to society as a whole. He examines the internal and the external sources and the existing incentives that explain different levels of development and the diffusion patterns of medical technology in the United States and other countries. He then raises questions about the changed direction of government commitments: from being prime supporters of biomedical research, development, and the diffusion of medical technology, to promoters of regulatory programs to ensure safety and efficacy, to proponents of controlling the diffusion and the application of medical technology. Banta is interested in the factors that encourage or inhibit the diffusion of technology and in the effects of these programs on people's health, the setting of priorities in health policy, and medical practices. How can the short-term importance of cost-benefit and cost-effectiveness analyses be balanced against the long-term importance of technology assessment? Can we afford to plan for health without acquiring a basic understanding of the factors that influence the practice of medicine? Will we negate or increase disparities and foster inequities without such knowledge?

From the perspective of economics, Jean François Lacronique and Simone Sandier discuss contradictory interpretations of technological innovation: Is it the cause or the victim of inflation? In particular, they examine technological progress in terms of the quality of medical care, technological effectiveness, economy, safety, convenience, and accessibility. By pointing to the dependence of French technological innovation on international influences, the authors critically inquire into the external and the internal factors that contribute to the expansion of technology and the roles played by different participants in this process. These participants include the research community, manufacturers, physicians as producers and consumers of innovation, the public as proponents of the best possible treatment, and, finally, financial organizations. They also focus attention on the trade-offs between market and control mechanisms.

Moving away from economic and public-policy issues (concerning the development and the diffusion of medical technology) to factors internal to the medical profession, Stuart S. Blume focuses on the impact of technological change on diagnostic medicine from a sociological point of view. In particular, he examines the criteria and the conceptions that guide the medical profession in assessing the value of new diagnostic technologies in the practice of medicine by drawing on three cases. Furthermore, the author raises the questions of a balance between "risk" and "accuracy"; the internal dynamics and the "self-generating" forces involved in adopting medical technology; diseconomies of scale; and, finally, the possibility of increasing inequalities in the receipt of medical care as a result of technological progress.

John M. C. Hattinga-Verschure broadens our view by going beyond the traditional conception of medical technology and care that restricts analyses of perceptions to those held by members of the professional subsystem. Instead, he develops a theoretical framework of care delivery that would require innovation in care and would result in mutual benefits to individuals, families, and communities. He then examines the distinct characteristics and the behavioral patterns involved in each kind of care and the interdependencies among them. Finally, he addresses how to overcome overmedicalization, overprofessionalization, and overinstitutionalization. Is a shift from the "medical model" to a "social model" of care necessary, and if so, is it sufficient?

Chapter 5

Public Policy and Medical Technology: Critical Issues Reconsidered

David Banta

This chapter will deal with the technology of medical care: the set of techniques, drugs, equipment, and procedures used by health-care professionals in delivering medical care to individuals. (77)[1] The technology of medical practice has changed dramatically in the past four decades, and there seems little doubt that many of these changes have proved valuable. Vaccines and antibiotics have helped empty the infectious disease wards since 1945, and methods are available to control a wide variety of diseases, including syphilis and gonorrhea, scarlet fever, cholera, yellow fever, typhoid fever, malaria, measles, rubella, smallpox, certain cancers, and certain endocrinologic and nutritional disorders. (10; 105, p. 35) The American Biology Council has issued a compilation of many medical innovations, introduced almost entirely in this century, that have contributed to human welfare. (2) Many of these innovations resulted from government policies designed to develop and use medical technology.

However, the evaluation of technological innovation began to change about a decade ago. Until the mid-sixties, it was generally assumed that all technology produced benefits in all sectors of the economy. However, as technology increased in scale rather than in scope, demonstrations of the utility of research and development were perceived as repetitious rather than innovative, and the negative effects of the use of technology became more apparent. Consequently, all science, including biomedical research, has come under scrutiny. A variety of commissions and other groups has begun to study biomedical research policies in the United States as well as in other countries. (12; 51; 79; 82; 91)

Feeding this increasing skepticism about technology is the growing recognition that the medical-care system has produced limited effects on the health of the population. McKeown has developed the case that dramatic improvements in mortality and morbidity in the last century, especially those resulting from the control of infectious diseases, stemmed in large part from broad societal changes, in particular, improvements in general nutrition. (64) This perspective informed the imaginative planning document of the Canadian government, which is based on the assumption that improvements in health will result from the execution of a plan that addresses four issues: genetic heritage, the environment (physical and social), life styles, and the medical-care system. (57)

During the past decade, the rapid rise in the cost of medical care has become the main political issue in the health arena in the United States. (23; 35) This rapid rise began in the late 1960s and has accelerated since 1967 at an annual rate of 10–15 percent. (39) Other countries have experienced even more rapid annual increases: 18 percent in Canada, 1974–1975; 19.3 percent in the Netherlands, 1970–1974; and 29 percent in Australia, 1975–1977. (85)

Many have identified medical technology as a contributor to the rising costs of medical care. (35; 36; 93; 110) Economists have estimated that technology accounts for up to half of the rise.[2] (1; 35; 110; 116) An examination of changes in the treatment of certain diseases has shown dramatic increases in costs. (97) Thomas coined the term *halfway technology* for technologies that are designed to compensate for disease or to postpone death but have yielded a limited impact in restoring health and are very expensive as well. (104) These technologies, which include organ transplantation and artificial organs, renal dialysis, the treatment of coronary artery disease, and most treatments for cancer, appear to be important contributors to medical-care costs. Dramatic cases of unproved, expensive technologies, such as gastric freezing for peptic ulcer in the 1960s (31) and the computed tomography scanner (7; 76; 125) and coronary bypass surgery in the 1970s (74; 83), have called into question the appropriateness of the processes involved in developing, diffusing, evaluating, and using medical technologies.

Pressure for change has come from the public, which expects ever-increasing improvements in medical care and ever-increasing rights to participate in making decisions about the processes of developing and using technology. (18, p. 5) Public concern has focused on expenditures for medical care under government programs, which have risen at nearly twice the rate of private expenditures. (39) Attitudes toward medical technology seem to be changing, leading to changes in policies directed toward developing, diffusing, evaluating, and using medical technologies. Irrespective of knowledge, decisions are made in the public arena, and policies have often been developed in the absence of informed projections of what their effects would be. (4; 123)

In this chapter, I will first sketch the development and the diffusion of medical technologies and then outline generic policies that have been formulated to deal with different stages in the processes of development and use. Without attempting a comprehensive analysis, I will review some evidence pertaining to the effects of some programs and will make comparisons with European systems designed to deal with the same processes. I will discuss some problems associated with processes and policies and will identify some important gaps in knowledge.

DEVELOPMENT AND DIFFUSION OF MEDICAL TECHNOLOGY

Medical advances rest in part on a foundation of knowledge about the biological mechanisms that underlie both the normal functioning of the human body and its malfunction in disease. When knowledge can be applied directly for the purposes of diagnosing, preventing, or curing disease, it can be termed medical technology. This technology is the result of a complex process of development. In a much quoted document, the President's Biomedical Research Panel delineated a number of steps in the process (82):

1. discovery, through research, of new knowledge and the relating of new knowledge to the existing base; [3]
2. translation of new knowledge, through applied research, into new technology and strategy for movement of discovery into health care;
3. validation of new technology through clinical trials;
4. determination of the safety and efficacy of new technology for widespread dissemination through demonstration projects;
5. education of the professional community in proper use of a new technology and of the lay community on the nature of these developments; and
6. skillful and balanced application of the new developments to the population.

The delineation of this sequence is important because it focuses attention on the fact that different policies should be devised for different stages of the process and indicates where intervention can occur. It is useful because it presents an orderly and comprehensible picture of the process, but it is unrealistic in the sense that it imposes structure on a process that is generally dynamic and disorderly. In fact, medical technology develops from processes in which basic research, applied research, development, and even diffusion progress simultaneously rather than sequentially. Subsequent steps reflect reactions to preceding ones, which affects the course of developments. Figure 5.1, a diagram showing the development of the cardiac pacemaker, illustrates this point.

The document fails to reflect the contributions of fields and disciplines not ordinarily considered by biomedical researchers. In particular, epidemiology often furnished knowledge of etiology and of effective preventive measures well before basic mechanisms of disease were understood. (17) The social sciences promise to provide much information of importance for the health of the population, not only with respect to such problems as mental illness and alcoholism but to such problems as the relation between stress and physical disease. (18)

Primarily as a result of extensive work in nonmedical areas, it has been found that the diffusion process usually follows an S-shaped or sigmoid curve in which the rate of adoption accelerates with the passage of time. (89) This time dimension is shown in Figure 5.2, a diagram showing the development and the diffusion of an idealized innovation. There are few quantitative studies of diffusion in the medical area, but the diffusion of some medical technologies follows the curve (Figure 5.3). (25; 89) The diffusion of other medical technologies does not, however, conform to the sigmoid curve. One major departure occurs when diffusion reaches a high rate almost immediately after the technology is introduced, represented in Figure 5.4 by the case of chemotherapy for leukemia. This so-called desperation reaction occurs in the absence of evidence about the efficacy of the innovation, apparently because of the provider's need to help a patient and their mutual desperation. (117) Generalizations about patterns of diffusion of medical technology seem unwarranted because of limited work in this area.

Whatever its initial pattern of diffusion, technology may eventually be partially or completely abandoned. Abandonment can occur when a rapidly-diffusing technology proves clinically to be of little use. A recent example is gastric freezing, which was widely diffused in the United States in the early 1960s but then ceased to be used. (31) Interestingly, abandonment had nothing to do with the formal evaluation of this technology, for clinical trials showing its lack of benefit were published after its disuse. Technologies can also be abandoned when a better technology becomes available, as happened with iron lungs after polio vaccine was

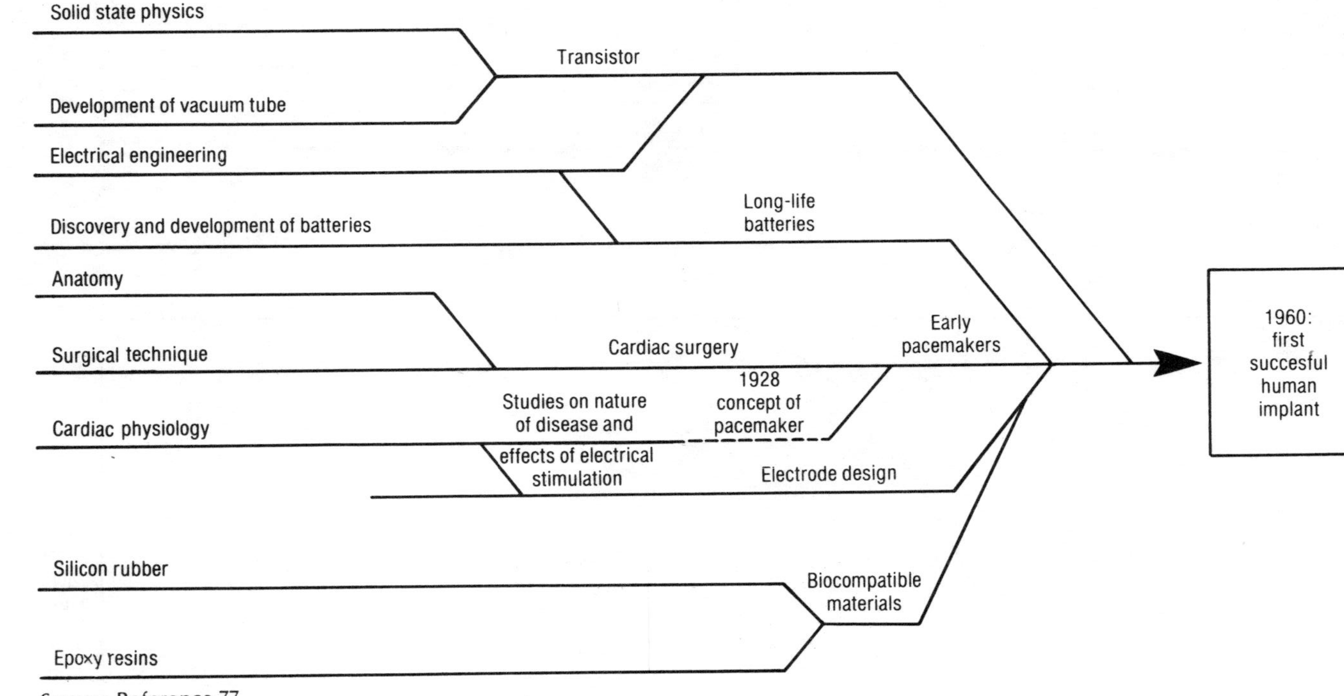

Source: Reference 77.

Figure 5.1. Development of the cardiac pacemaker.

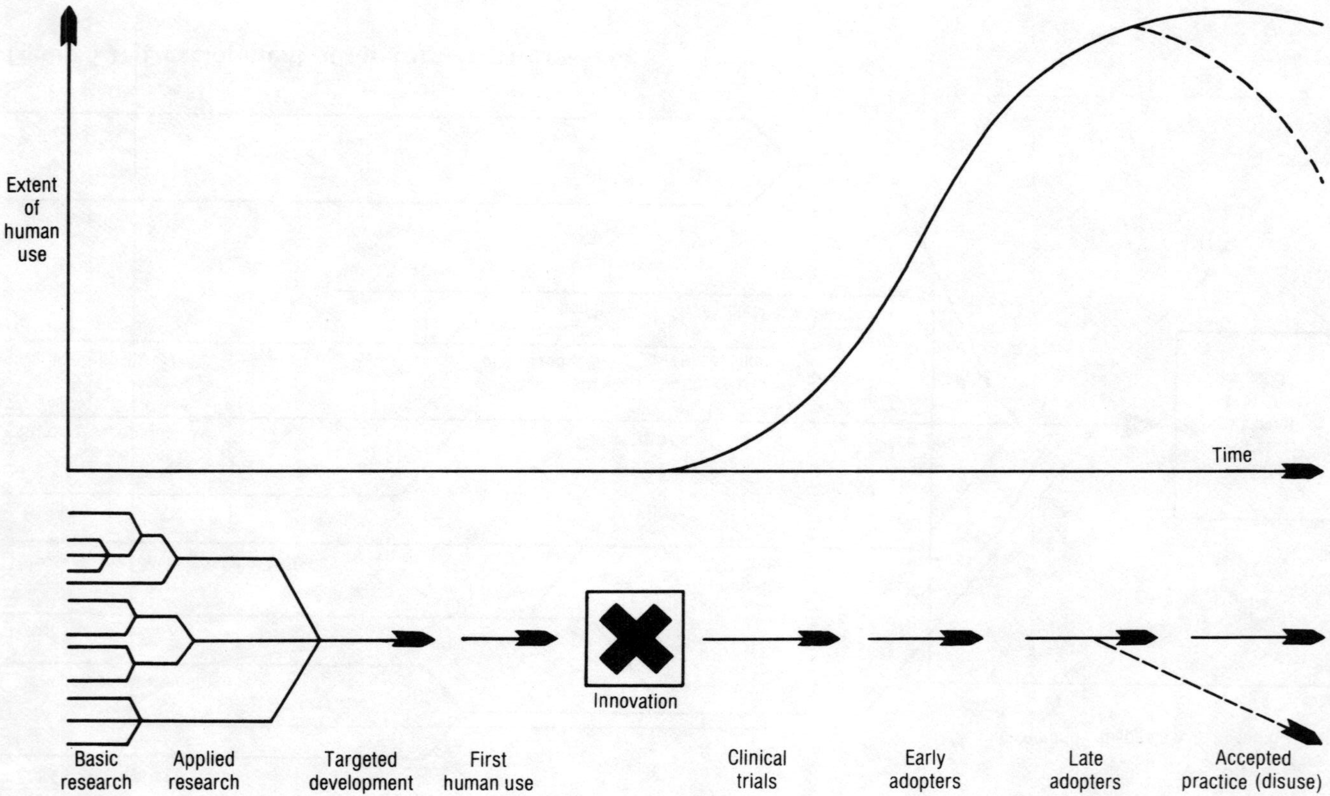

Source: Reference 77.

Figure 5.2. A scheme for development and diffusion of medical technologies.

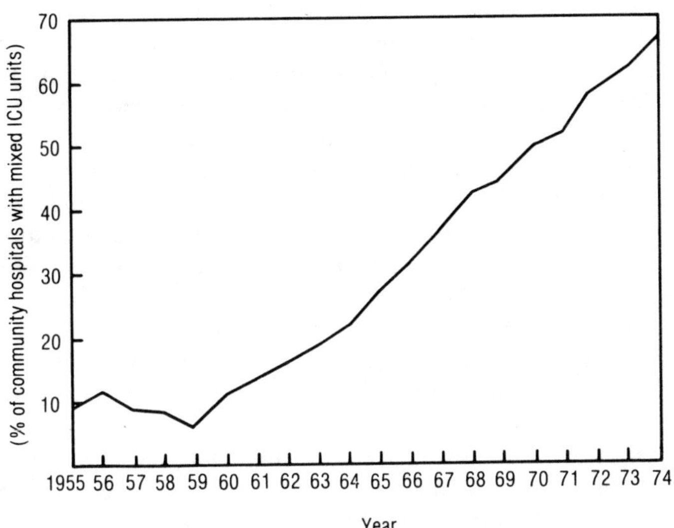

Source: References 89 and 117.

Figure 5.3. The diffusion of some medical technologies.

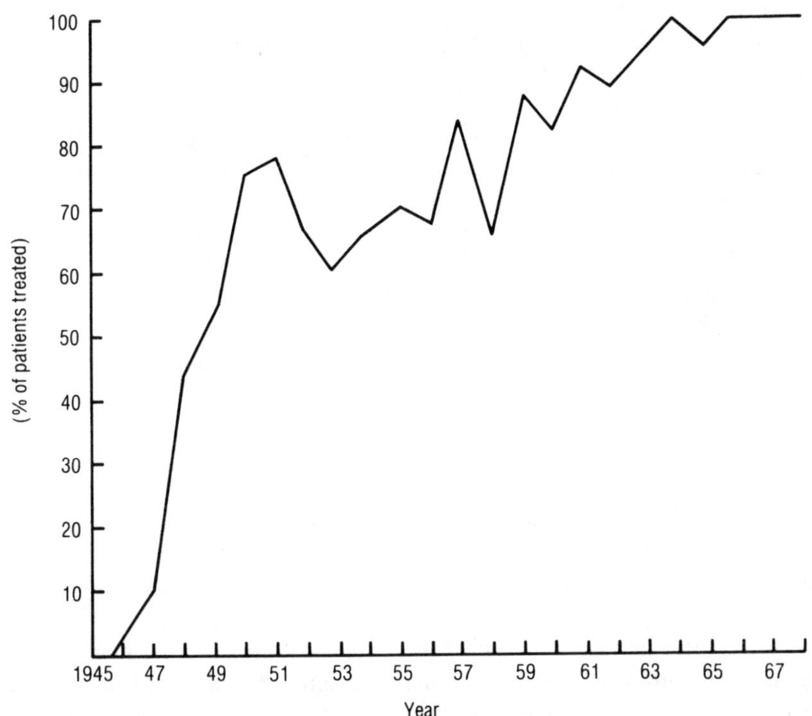

Source: Reference 117.

Figure 5.4. Chemotherapy for leukemia.

developed (105, p. 36) or with pneumoencephalography after the development of computed tomography head scanning. (125) Hiatt has produced a long list of technologies that used to be widespread but were virtually abandoned because of the lack of efficacy. (48)

There are inevitable time lags between the conception of an idea or an innovation and the introduction of the corresponding technology. If the interval is short, the technology might not have been completely developed or thoroughly tested, as happened with X-rays. If the lag is long, patients who might benefit are needlessly deprived of therapy. (78) Several studies have found that median lags between the conception of an idea and the availability of the medical technology were ten years or less. (9; 22) Another study reported time lags to be shorter for drugs. (62, p. 181)

Unfortunately, there is no reason to think that such time lags can be shortened appreciably without sacrificing appropriate caution. Serious lags do result, however, from the delayed adoption of available technologies. Studies evaluating the quality of care indicate that the most appropriate diagnostic or therapeutic procedure is not often used in medical practice. For example, drug treatment for hypertension is known to prevent disease and disability in patients who suffer from severe high blood pressure (108), yet surveys have shown that 50 percent of hypertensives in the United States were unaware that they had elevated blood pressure and only about fourteen percent were being adequately treated.[4] (111)

In general, the incentives in the United States are skewed toward the premature acceptance of technologies, which seems to be the major problem. (34; 40; 118) There are few sellers of either medical services or medical technology and many barriers to entry. The public is ignorant of what is available and lacks the expertise needed to make rational choices. Physicians have been granted extraordinary powers to make decisions about the treatment of their patients and about the technology used by the institutions in which they work. (70, p. 34) And the widespread third-party insurance coverage in the United States and the comprehensive systems of other countries have removed most financial barriers against the introduction of technology. Physicians want to provide every possible kind of therapy for their patients (48; 104), and institutions, especially hospitals, compete to be the most innovative. Thus technical innovations diffuse rapidly in the United States as well as in other countries.

Public intervention in the processes of developing, diffusing, and using medical technology has led to policies designed to address the problems of cost, the effective use of resources, and the evaluation of health-care systems.

PUBLIC POLICY TOWARD MEDICAL TECHNOLOGY

Federal laws and agencies only partially express public policies. In the United States, private organizations play a large part in controlling the health-care system and in many cases use the authority that has been delegated to them. The investment in developing technology made by private industry is substantial. (60) Almost all medical insurance is either private or is administered by private organizations. States and municipalities have also enacted laws that in some cases parallel federal laws and in other cases conflict with them. However, this section will present a discussion of only the federal government's role in overseeing the health-care system.

Within the federal government, many departments play roles in the health-care system. The Department of Defense and the Veterans Administration operate large medical-care systems. However, the Department of Health, Education and Welfare plays the largest role in attempting to rationalize and control the "pluralistic" health-care system, which will be the focus of this discussion. Table 5.1 summarizes relevant programs in the department.

TECHNOLOGY DEVELOPMENT

In the United States, as in all industrialized countries, the government has assumed major responsibility for the support of biomedical research and the development of medical technology. (77; 87) Government investment, particularly in basic research, is rationalized on the grounds that the private sector limits its investments in inventions and research. Underinvestment exists because private firms cannot retain all the profit from innovations. (87) In 1975 the total investment in biomedical research and development in the United States was about $4.6 billion, $2.8 billion, or 60.8 percent, of which was expended by the federal government. About two-thirds of the federal amount was administered by the National Institutes of Health. (28, pp. 393–394) The priorities for biomedical research in the United States are set in an exceedingly complex manner. Congress controls budget priorities but delegates considerable discretionary authority to the National Institutes of Health. (82; 99; 103) However, the dependence on researcher-initiated projects (research developed through the initiative of individuals) limits flexibility and planning. In the past few years, NIH has been subject to considerable pressure to plan its research activities more efficiently and to address real health needs through the development of technology. (100) The burden of illness, an adequate science base, researchers' curiosity, and the public perceptions of need have all been suggested as criteria for investment (18, pp. 20–24, 87; 119), but little guidance has been given to enable NIH to rank these criteria.

Table 5.1. Technology Development and Use: Formal Programs of the Department of Health, Education and Welfare

Stage of Development	*Function*	*Agency(s) or Program(s)*
Basic research	Support of research; planning of research	National Institutes of Health; small investments by others
Applied research	Support and planning of research	National Institutes of Health; several other agencies; several other departments
Clinical trials	Test safety; test efficacy; protect human subjects	National Institutes of Health; small investments by others
Assure efficacy and safety of drugs and devices	Approval for market; control procedures used for testing; some post-marketing surveillance	Food and Drug Administration
Assess social impact	Cost benefit; cost effectiveness; technology assessment	National Center for Health Services Research; National Institutes of Health (limited)
Diffusion	Control of drugs and devices	Food and Drug Administration (See above.)
Diffusion	Encourage distribution	National Institutes of Health (limited)
Diffusion	Control distribution; certificate of need	Health Resources Administration (Bureau of Health Planning)
Widespread use	Reimbursement; define benefit package; set reimbursement levels	Medicare (elderly); Medicaid (poor)
Widespread use	Ensure appropriate use	Certification programs; Professional Standards Review Organizations (PSRO)
Widespread use	Monitor practice	Professional Standards Review Organizations (limited)

Note: As one proceeds downward, the federal role generally becomes weaker.

TECHNOLOGY EVALUATION AND TRANSFER

No federal agency has been given formal responsibility for the overall evaluation and efficient transfer (diffusion) of medical technology. The NIH, as the major supporter of research and development, funds a certain number of studies concerning the efficacy and the safety of technologies. In 1975 NIH expended about $100 million on 755 clinical trials related to efficacy. Of that total, 535 trials tested drugs either in isolation or in combination with other methods of treatment. However, only 25 trials evaluated surgical procedures. Very few examined the efficacy of screening, early diagnosis, or primary prevention. (72) NIH has supported important clinical trials, including ongoing tests of tonsillectomy (80) and radical mastectomy. (33) But the institution has not taken an active role in evaluating technologies in widespread use. (18, p. 36)

The Food and Drug Administration (FDA) also plays an important role in evaluating technology, which will be described below.

Other agencies of the Department of Health, Education and Welfare and other federal departments fund clinical trials. For example, the Maternal and Child Health Program (44) and the Veterans Administration (107; 108) have funded important clinical trials. A few cost-effectiveness or cost-benefit studies have also been supported, especially by the National Center for Health Services Research. However, these efforts are small in size. Legislation considered during 1978 mandated the establishment of a National Center for the Evaluation of Medical Technology in the Department of Health, Education and Welfare.

REGULATION OF MEDICAL TECHNOLOGY

Problems pertaining to the development, the diffusion, and the use of medical technologies, as well as those related to risk, the lack of technological efficacy, and rising health-care costs have stimulated a variety of regulatory programs. This section contains brief descriptions of some of these programs.

Assurance of Safety and Efficacy

The manufacture and the distribution of drugs are vested in the private sector in most Western countries, and that sector is heavily oriented to profits. Thus within that sector of the health-care system, such problems as fostering overuse and the marketing of drugs of limited efficacy or those that produce high levels of risk have led to regulatory controls. The Food and Drug Administration (FDA) is required by law to regulate production processes and determine that a drug is efficacious and safe before it can be marketed. Under this program, a company wishing to market a drug must submit evidence from well-controlled clinical trials of the safety and the efficacy of these technologies.

The FDA also has long-standing statutory authority to ensure the safety of radiological equipment. It promulgates standards for X-ray equipment and enforces various programs to ensure that standards are met and that the radiation exposure of the population is minimized.

Since 1976, the FDA has been given authority to regulate the safety and the efficacy of medical devices. The law under which this authority was delegated was stimulated by examples of death or morbidity resulting from the use of badly-made devices. Although the law is still being implemented, it is clear that it will exert considerable impact on this aspect of medical technology.

Controlling Diffusion

Concerns generated by rising costs of health care led to the 1974 health planning law. Perhaps the most important section of the law mandates local agencies and 50 state agencies to review and approve institutional capital investments through a certificate-of-need process. This law supplements the certificate-of-need laws of more than 20 states and replaces Section 1122 of the Social Security Act, the purpose of which was to control institutional capital investments. Capital investments over $150,000 are covered. Thus the computed tomography (CT) scanner, which costs several hundred thousand dollars, is subject to review, as are hospital beds. Proposed amendments to the law could lower the financial limit and extend the review to noninstitutional settings.[5]

Controlling the Use of Medical Technology

The use of technology can be regulated directly, for example, a physician's prescription or regulated indirectly, for example, insurance schemes that will not pay for the use of technology. Regulating fees or charges is also a form of regulating technology.

The reimbursement system in the United States has so far been little used to promote the wise use of technology. The widespread coverage for hospital care and the spotty coverage for outpatient and preventive care have accorded primacy to the hospital sector. Medicare, the major government health-insurance program, pays physicians "usual and customary" fees and reimburses hospitals for their costs of providing care. Both methods have proved inflationary. Physicians function in hospitals where they can use technologies without incurring financial risk. However, during the past several years, the administrators of the Medicare program have begun to examine certain medical procedures to ascertain whether they are outmoded and if so, to reject claims for payment. They are examining payment for CT scanning and as late as the spring of 1978, were not paying for body scanning on the grounds that it was not a necessary technology.

In 1972 the Professional Standards Review Organization (PSRO) program was established to ensure that payment for services under the Medicare and Medicaid programs would only be made when the services performed were deemed necessary. The law established 203 organizations directed by physicians. PSROs review services under federal reimbursement programs. So far they have focused on hospital-bed use but are beginning to consider whether surgical procedures should be reviewed. The national PSRO program is considering reviewing the use of diagnostic technologies, especially laboratory testing and CT scanning.

EVALUATION OF PROGRAMS REGULATING MEDICAL TECHNOLOGY

The Food and Drug Administration

The FDA program to regulate the introduction of drugs has generated controversy. Criticism continues to be directed against the "drug lag" that is alleged to result from FDA procedures that keep useful drugs off the market an inordinately long time and the costs of such a lag in both human and financial terms. Peltzman examined the question of lag by comparing drug innovation in pre-1962 and post-1962 periods. He found a large decrease in the introduction of drugs in the latter period. Crossnational studies (26; 42; 112; 113; 114; 115) demonstrate that the United States tends to lag behind such countries as Britain, France, Germany, and Italy in the introduction of drugs. De Haen, however, has shown that a drug lag exists to some extent in each country. (26) To the charge that the United States lags behind the industrialized countries of Western Europe (58), FDA spokesmen have argued that the drug lag has not affected the rate of important therapeutic advances. (101) Furthermore, they contend, such important advances are expedited through FDA processes. (32; 124) The extensive literature on the question of drug lag does not resolve the question of whether the FDA program benefits or harms the aggregate health of the public. (95)

The FDA program to protect the public from inappropriate X-ray exposure has apparently not caused lags and therefore has not generated controversy. The program has not been subjected to formal evaluation.

Because the medical-devices law was enacted recently, its effectiveness cannot be evaluated. Nevertheless, speculations about its potential adverse effects on innovation and its potential beneficial effects on efficacy and safety have been published. (5; 8)

The Health Planning Program

The 1974 health planning law is also too recent to evaluate, but some studies have projected its effects. The general experience with regulatory programs in the United States suggests that the program may protect established hospitals from competition and may be controlled by the powerful interests that it is intended to regulate. (45; 75) Several studies evaluated the effects of previous planning programs, including state certificate of need programs, and found that they curtailed bed expansion. (11; 47; 90) The most widely-quoted study examined the effects of certificates-of-need from 1968 to 1972 and found some curtailment of bed expansion. However, the study found no reduction in cost because there appeared to be a shift in hospital investments from beds to facilities and equipment. (94) Another study found that a certificate-of-need law was negatively related to the adoption of X-ray, cobalt, and radium therapy but was not related to the adoption of such services as intensive care, open heart surgery, and diagnostic nuclear medicine. (25)

The passage of the 1974 health planning law and such developments as National Guidelines for Health Planning (29) are attempts to make health planning more effective and thus make these findings of limited usefulness in understanding the future effects of health-planning programs. A large study is under way to examine the effects of certificates of need. It is focused on cases of more recent origin and is much more detailed than studies conducted in the past. (24)

The Professional Standards Review Organizations

The PSRO program is still in the process of implementation—by the fall of 1977, no local PSRO had been certified as an operating agency, and more than 20 of the 203 PSRO areas did not even have a PSRO in the "planning" stage. Nonetheless, a few studies have suggested what later evaluations may show. An evaluation of the performance of 18 selected

PSROs during 1974–1977 found no statistically-significant effect on hospital use or admissions rates. (46) Indeed, the incentives of the PSRO program tend to favor quality of care over cost containment (16), and there were some indications that PSROs improved clinical and administrative deficiencies of care. (46) Furthermore, some individual PSROs generated economies in the use of hospital beds to pay for themselves.

Further evaluations must await the implementation of the program and perhaps the clarification of its goals.

Final Comments on Regulatory Programs

This selective review can cover only a limited number of programs designed to affect the diffusion and the use of medical technologies. Policies directed toward malpractice, manpower development, the structural approval of plans for facilities, and so forth would, of course, be described in a full discussion.

All of these programs are hindered by a lack of information about the costs, risks, and benefits of medical technology. (7; 48; 69; 125)

It is important to recognize that the programs described are limited in their mandates and scope. The FDA controls the marketing of drugs and devices but seldom intervenes after the initial decision to allow marketing. The health-planning program is decentralized and exerts authority over a limited number of technologies that require large capital investments. Reimbursement decisions are more comprehensive in scope but are not generally used to exercise control. The PSRO program reviews only hospital services provided to beneficiaries of federal programs through a decentralized, physician-controlled mechanism. Thus although coverage is generally spotty and weak, it should become stronger and more comprehensive in the future. (49)

It is also striking how little is known about the effects of these programs. Virtually nothing is known that could answer the question of whether the health of the population has been improved or harmed by the implementation of these policies.

SOME INTERNATIONAL COMPARISONS

Technology Development

As in the United States, industrialized countries have instituted mechanisms to support biomedical research and the development of technology. (79; 87) But the process of establishing program priorities has not been described. (87) Klein has commented that biomedical research priorities in Britain have tended to be shaped by the interests of the research community rather than by knowledge derived from an appraisal of what kinds of research would yield the greatest dividend to the community at large. (56)

The Evaluation of Medical Technology

Evaluations of medical technology are carried out in government agencies. Britain has carried out several useful, controlled clinical trials. (20) Sweden has also supported clinical trials and other evaluations of medical technologies. (52; 74) In both Britain and Belgium, operations research has become a field of inquiry. (55) France has supported several studies of the economics of health advances and the cost benefits of certain technologies. (14, pp. 190–210) Although private organizations have made significant contributions (66; 67; 68), their investments have been small.

It is not possible to make country-by-country comparisons of the number or the quality of the studies that have been conducted. The state of general knowledge suggests that no country is doing well. Klein has noted that in England, as in the United States, consensus on the part of physicians often substitutes for the evaluation of goals and public involvement. (56) The same observation could be made about Sweden. (15, pp. 46–47)

Blanpain stated that the mandatory, systematic appraisal of diagnostic and therapeutic procedures has repeatedly been proposed in Europe. (15, p. 23) It is not known how often countries use evaluations of technology in policymaking, for such descriptions as Sweden's experience with coronary artery surgery (74) are rare.

Regulation of Drugs

Most countries have imposed controls over the introduction of drugs similar to those of the United Sates, although controls over production, as in Norway, appear to be more limited. (88) In West Germany tests used for verifying safety were not as rigorous as those used in the United States (88) until 1978, when a program modeled on the FDA's was implemented. However, important constraints are applied to drugs. Ministries of health often issue lists of compounds that may be imported or sold, for example, Norway recently authorized the sale of only 2,000 drugs. (88) In Britain there is a recommended list of products that can be dispensed under the National Health Services. Nonlisted products must be paid for by patients. (88)

Approval of Facilities

Hospital construction and, to some extent, other capital investments have been subject to government controls in West European countries. (37; 88) Hospital standards are developed centrally in Britain, the Netherlands, and France. (63; 88) France has a National Committee that must approve the purchase of major equipment. (37) In Canada, the federal government exerts budgetary pressure to limit facilities, and global-hospital budgeting and capital controls operate through the budget process at the provincial level. (59, p. 22) West Germany has a separate capital budget controlled at the state level. (37) However, although the existence of excess hospital beds has been perceived as a serious problem in both the United States and Canada, this perception has not prevailed in Western Europe, which has a larger number of beds per capita. (88; 126)

Regulation of the Use of Technology

The German sickness funds carry out computerized reviews of each physician's practice, including the number of prescriptions issued, the number of lab tests conducted per case, the rates of certain surgical procedures performed, and so forth. (88) In Canada, each province has a utilization-review mechanism, and although these reviews are primarily oriented toward uncovering overbilling and fraud, several provinces are developing more sophisticated reviews, including patterns of practice by diagnosis. (59, p. 22) Fees are sometimes set to encourage or discourage certain activities when fees for service constitute the method of payment, as in West Germany and Canada. (88)

Comments on the International Experience

This review indicates that the programs of other countries parallel those of the United States. The problems are often the same, and the processes and policies are similar. However, little seems to be known about the effects of the policies, and few international comparisons have been made outside the area of drugs. It is worth noting that West European countries generally seem to take a more skeptical stance than does the United States regarding some medical technology. An example is the case of coronary artery surgery. (83)

GENERIC PROBLEMS AND ISSUES

The question of allocating resources to support research has been alluded to, as has been the problem of planning for the use of these resources. In addition to focusing on the question of how to set priorities, one could criticize under investment in newer or less traditional areas of health research. In particular, behavioral and social science, environmental and occupational health, epidemiology, mental health, and prevention are areas that have been identified as underemphasized in health research. (18, p. 23; 51) Evaluating products (the technologies) through clinical trials or other methods has also been underemphasized.

At the stage of diffusion, efficacy, safety, and use have often not been effectively demonstrated. No federal agency in the United States has an explicit charge to carry out this task, and investments are small. Furthermore, information on efficacy and safety is seldom synthesized by expert groups, and so regulatory authorities make decisions arbitrarily or on the basis of clinical opinion. (78) Nevertheless, in the United States at least, health-planning agencies appear to be eager to obtain information about the efficacy of some technologies such as the CT scanner. (125)

NIH identified a series of problems in the transfer of technology that seems to have international validity: (21)

1. Formal processes are lacking to ensure "systematic identification and evaluation of clinically relevant research information and its effective transfer to the health care community."
2. There are problems in application: "Some validated interventions may diffuse too slowly through the health delivery system; others, in the absence of validation and consensus, may be applied prematurely or inappropriately."
3. "Neither Congress nor the Executive Branch has assigned specific agency responsibilities for dealing with these health spectrum deficiencies." (73)

Although the international diffusion of technology has received little attention, it is sometimes of great importance. By the end of 1977, the United States had bought about 500 CT scanners made by EMI Ltd., a British company, for about $200 million.

These problems suggest the need for imposing more controls (15, pp. 24–25) through the reimbursement system or through direct regulation to "assure that only adequately assessed technologies are disseminated" (18, p. 44) and to facilitate the diffusion and the use of worthwhile technologies. The more formal evaluation of technologies before they come into general use is one approach that appears to be promising. (3; 6; 78)

SOME IMPORTANT GAPS IN KNOWLEDGE

Few studies of the processes and programs described above have been conducted. There is certainly a need to learn how to derive maximum benefits from investments in health research. The contribution of basic biomedical research, compared with other possible investments, is not known. (18, p. 15) Indeed, the role of research in generating useful knowledge, as well as how the dissemination of such information changes medical practice from year to year, is poorly understood. (27; 93; 109) The efficacy and safety of any medical technology cannot be determined from the professional literature because the necessary studies have not been done. (78) We do not know how to ensure the application of efficacious technologies such as drug therapy for hypertension. And the effectiveness of different methods and systems for delivering health care and influencing the health of the population has seldom been compared. In fact, the methodology for doing such studies has not been developed. (30)

The most rigorous method for determining the efficacy and safety of medical technology is the controlled clinical trial. However, clinical trials are difficult to organize and carry out. Because large population groups are required to demonstrate a statistically-significant effect on the status of health, clinical trials would be both difficult to carry out and very expensive to conduct. Another major problem is that although reducing mortality and improving physical morbidity are not the only objectives sought, other outcomes, such as social functioning, are very difficult to measure. (78) Thus there is a need to devise an effective alternative to the controlled clinical trial. (19; 38; 120; 121; 122)

Diffusion is another critical stage in the process of developing technology that has been little studied. Studies indicate that physicians are influenced most by their own experience and that of their respected colleagues. (43; 53; 96) Other sources of information, such as advertising campaigns, the technical literature, and programs of continuing education, can be important but seem to be secondary in impact. Studies of institutions suggest that large hospitals that offer comprehensive services and university-affiliated hospitals adopt innovations faster than other hospitals. (40; 54; 84) The incidence of physicians in an area has been related to rapid diffusion and adoption. (25) However, few studies included variables of importance to the determination of public policy, such as the political climate, community decision-making patterns, and the nature and the number of interorganizational programs. (54) As noted above, few studies have examined the effects of such public policies as health-planning and reimbursement programs. (71)

Factors that influence the use of medical technology need to be better understood. Such understanding can only come from health-services research. As a report of the President's Science Advisory Committee stated:

> The focus in health services R&D is on making biomedical knowledge available to treat, control and eliminate disease and to restore function or to minimize disability, rather than on the development of new knowledge. Therefore, biomedical research and health services research are complementary, although at times the boundaries between them are blurred. The success of the former implies the need for the latter. If we fail to invest adequately in health services research to improve the availability of knowledge developed in the laboratory, we cannot realize the full benefits of our investment in biomedical research. (50)

Despite this recognition, health-services research has been underfunded in the United States (4; 123) and is underdeveloped in most of Europe. (14) However, worldwide interest in developing comprehensive and integrated approaches to health problems through better planning and coordination (13; 30; 67; 98) should promote the growth of this field. (67)

A related and important innovation is the development of data systems that can evaluate individual providers and institutions. (106) The Nordic countries have apparently achieved the most success in developing systems for acquiring information on which to base decisions about the health system. (66) Given the fact that demonstrating the efficacy and the safety of a medical technology is only the first step in applying it to improve health, these data systems are critical for both monitoring performance and for generating research on factors that encourage or inhibit the use of certain technologies.

SUMMARY AND CONCLUSIONS

As stated in the planning documents of many countries (30, p. 44), the major goal of the medical-care system is to improve health. (70, p. 54) However, the decade of the 1970s developed the perception that medical technology has not always been beneficial and that even when it appears to be, it may not be worth the cost in both human and financial terms. All medical technology is now subject to scrutiny. Rising costs have forced the awareness that rationing is necessary (48) and have led to the formulation of policies concerning medical innovation, ranging from changing priorities for biomedical research to controlling the use of technology. The immediate prospect is for the imposition of more controls and greater regulation of technology. (49)

This prospect makes ever more acute the need for research concerning the development and the use of medical technologies. High priority should be accorded to research in the following areas:

1. Research on research, development, and diffusion, with an emphasis on diffusion;
2. research on an alternative system of providing medical care directed toward evaluating its effectiveness in preventing and treating disease;
3. research on specific technologies, focusing on those that are in wide use, that are applied or will be applied to a disease that is prevalent, that are very expensive, or that involve safety risks; good candidates can be found in obstetrics, diagnostic medicine, and surgery. Ascertaining the uses of technologies should be the most important immediate outcome of such research. Cost-benefit and cost-effectiveness analyses are of short-term importance; technology assessment is of long-term importance; (3)
4. research on methods: methods of evaluating medical technologies are especially needed.

The dynamic that conduces to the proliferation of technology in medicine, the growth in chronic diseases, the prevalence of disease in the community, and the high expectations of medical practitioners will inevitably increase pressures on health systems. The pressures seem to explain the upsurge of interest in comprehensive health planning throughout the world. However, planning made without the knowledge of what medical-care practices affect health outcomes could increase disparities and foster inequities. And it is unfortunately true that little evidence has been generated about which health-care practices affect health. (20; 69; 78)

The challenge has been well stated by the director of the World Health Organization, who suggested that the design of a national health system might be based on responses to four questions:

1. Is it possible to assign health resources within a country on a problem-solving basis, using different mixes of preventive, curative, promotive, and rehabilitative actions?
2. What medical interventions are truly effective and specific for prevention, treatment, or rehabilitation, as measured in objective terms?

3. Can such medical interventions and the risk groups to which they should be applied be described objectively and in such a manner that the amount of skill and knowledge required for their application can be assessed?
4. Is it possible to design a health care establishment to carry out the above tasks which will result in the most meaningful interventions reaching the greatest proportion of persons at risk, as early as possible, at the least cost, and in an acceptable manner? (61)

NOTES

1. Technology is defined as science or knowledge applied to a purpose. This definition is broader than the common usage of applying the term only to medical equipment. The definition is broad enough to accommodate the perspectives of a variety of disciplines, including economists' perception of a production function in health care, that is, defining the physical relationship between inputs and outputs. Medical technology includes the systems within which care is delivered and such supports as computers. This chapter will deal with those kinds of technology only indirectly.
2. These estimates are not based on the actual costs of technology as defined in this paper but on proxy measures. In particular, it has been observed that changes in hospital prices account for about half of the rise in hospital costs. The remainder is considered to represent additional equipment, supplies, and labor and has been labeled the technology factor. (37) The true contribution of technology to rising costs may be less than 30 percent. (116)
3. It is worth noting that advances in medical technology often draw on bodies of knowledge not usually thought of as biomedical, such as electronics and engineering. (99)
4. This fact led to the development of programs to improve the situation. Some data suggest that changes have occurred, although, at most, 29 percent of hypertensives had been adequately treated.
5. Many CT scanners were purchased for office settings, especially after health-planning agencies attempted to constrain their institutional diffusion.

REFERENCES

1. Altman, S. H., and Wallack, S. S. "Technology on Trial—Is It the Culprit Behind Rising Health Costs? The Case For and Against." Presented at the Sun Valley Forum on National Health, Sun Valley, Idaho, August 1–5, 1977.
2. American Biology Council. *Contributions of the Biological Sciences to Human Welfare. Federation Proceedings,* vol. 31, 1972.
3. Arnstein, S. R. "Technology Assessment: Opportunities and Obstacles." In *IEEE Transactions on Systems, Man and Cybernetics. SMC* 7: 571, 1977.
4. Banta, H. D., and Bauman, P. "Health Services Research and Health Policy." *J. Comm. Health* 2: 121, 1976.
5. Banta, H. D., Brown, S., and Behney, C. "Implications of the 1976 Medical Devices Legislation." *Man and Medicine,* forthcoming.

6. Banta, H. D., and Sanes, J. R. "Assessing the Social Impacts of Medical Technologies." *J. Comm. Health* 3: 245, 1978.
7. ———. "How the CAT Got out of the Bag." Presented at the conference on Health-Care Technology and the Quality of Care, Boston University Health Policy Center, Boston, Mass., November 19–20, 1976.
8. Baram, M. "Medical Device Legislation and the Development and Diffusion of Health Technology." Presented at the conference on Health-Care Technology and the Quality of Care, Boston University Health Policy Center, Boston, Mass., November 19–20, 1976.
9. Battelle Columbus Laboratories. "Analysis of Selected Biomedical Research Programs." In *Report of the President's Biomedical Research Panel,* Washington, D.C.: Department of Health, Education, and Welfare, 1976. App. B, p. 35 (DHEW Publication No. OS 75-502).
10. Bennett, I. "Technology as a Shaping Force." *Daedalus* 106: 125, 1977.
11. Bicknell, W., and Walsh, D. "Certificate of Need: The Massachusetts Experience." *N.E.J.M.* 292: 1054, 1975.
12. *Biomedical Science and Its Administration* (The "Wooldridge Report"). Washington, D.C.: The White House, February 1965.
13. Black, D. "What Should Now Be Done by Government?" *Proc. Roy. Soc. Med.* 67: 1306, 1974.
14. Blanpain, J., and Delesie, L. *Community Health Investment, Health Services Research in Belgium, France, Federal German Republic and the Netherlands.* London: Oxford University Press, 1976.
15. Blanpain, J., et al. *International Approaches to Health Resources Development for National Health Programs, Executive Summary of the Study.* Hyattsville, Md.: Health Resources Administration, Department of Health, Education, and Welfare, 1976.
16. Blumstein, J. "The Role of PSROs in Hospital Cost Containment." In M. Zubkoff, I. Raskin, and R. Hanft, eds., *Hospital Cost Containment: Selected Notes for Future Policy.* New York: Prodist, 1978, pp. 461–485.
17. Breslow, L. *Testimony on Basic Issues in Biomedical Research* Before the U.S. Senate Subcommittee on Health, Committee on Labor and Public Welfare, Washington, D.C., June 17, 1976.
18. Brown, S. *Policy Issues in the Health Sciences.* Washington, D.C.: Institute of Medicine, National Academy of Sciences, 1977.
19. Bunker, J. P., Barnes, B. A., and Mosteller, F. eds. *Costs, Risks, and Benefits of Surgery.* New York: Oxford University Press, 1977.
20. Cochrane, A. L. *Effectiveness and Efficiency.* London: Burgess & Son Ltd. (Nuffield Provincial Hospitals Trust), 1972.
21. Cochrane, A. "Some Reflections." In G. McLachlan, ed. *A Question of Quality? Roads to Assurance in Medical Care.* London: Oxford University Press, 1976, p. 257.
22. Comroe, J. H. "Lags Between Initial Discovery and Clinical Application to Cardiovascular Pulmonary Medicine and Surgery." In *Report of the President's Biomedical Research Panel.* Washington, D.C.: Department of Health, Education, and Welfare, 1976. Appendix B, p. 1. (DHEW Publication No. OS 75-502.)

23. Council on Wage and Price Stability. *The Complex Puzzle of Rising Health Care Costs: Can the Private Sector Fit It Together.* Washington, D.C.: Executive Office of the President, 1976.
24. Cromwell, J. *Evaluation of Effects of Certificate of Need Programs.* Contract No. HRA 231-77-0114, National Center for Health Services Research. Rockville, Md.: Department of Health, Education, and Welfare, 1977.
25. Cromwell, J., et al. *Incentives and Decisions Underlying Hospitals' Adoption and Utilization of Major Capital Equipment.* Boston, Mass.: Abt Associates, Inc., 1975.
26. De Haen, P. "The Drug Lag—Does It Exist in Europe?" *Drug Intelligence and Clinical Pharmacy* 9: 144, 1975.
27. Department of Health, Education, and Welfare. *Forward Plan for Health, FY 1978–82.* Washington, D.C.: U.S. Government Printing Office, 1976, pp. 95–96.
28. ———. *Health, United States, 1976–1977.* Washington, D.C.: U.S. Government Printing Office, 1977.
29. ———. "National Guidelines for Health Planning." *Federal Register* 43: 13040, March 28, 1978.
30. ———. *Papers on the National Health Guidelines: Baselines for Setting Health Goals and Standards.* Washington, D.C.: U.S. Government Printing Office, 1976. (DHEW Publication No. HRA 76-640.)
31. Fineberg, H. V. "Gastric Freezing, A Study of Diffusion of a Medical Innovation." Prepared for the Commitee on Technology and Health Care, National Academy of Sciences, Washington, D.C., August 1977.
32. Finkel, M. "FDA Implementing Plans to Cut by One or Two Years New-Drug Approval Lag," *Medical Tribune* 14: 1, 1973.
33. Fisher, B. "Primary Therapy of Breast Cancer: A Report." In *Report to the Profession—Breast Cancer.* Washington, D.C.: National Cancer Institute, National Institutes of Health, 1974, pp. 157–170.
34. Fuchs, V. R. "Health Care and the U.S. Economic System, An Essay in Abnormal Physiology." *Milbank Mem. Fund Quart.* L: 211, 1972.
35. Gaus, G. *Biomedical Research and Health Care Costs.* Testimony Before the President's Biomedical Research Panel, Washington, D.C., September 29, 1975.
36. Gaus, C. R., and Cooper, B. S. "Controlling Health Technology." Presented at the Sun Valley Forum on National Health, Sun Valley, Idaho, August 1–5, 1977.
37. Gaus, C. R., and Cooper, B. S. "Technology and Medicare: Alternatives for Change." Presented at the conference on Health Care Technology and the Quality of Care, Boston University Health Policy Center, Boston, Mass., November 19–20, 1976. (to be published in 1978 by Aspen Systems, Inc.)
38. Gehan, E., and Freireich, E. "Nonrandomized Control in Cancer Clinical Trials." *N.E.J.M.* 290: 198, 1974.
39. Gibson, R. M., and Mueller, M. S. "National Health Expenditures, Fiscal Year 1976." *Social Security Bulletin* 40: 3–22, 1977, and personal communication, R. M. Gibson, 1978.

40. Gordon, G., and Fisher, G. L., eds. *The Diffusion of Medical Technology,* Cambridge, Mass.: Ballinger Publishing Co., 1975.
41. Grabowski, H. G., and Vernon, J. M. "Innovation and Invention, Consumer Protection Regulation in Ethical Drugs." *American Economic Association Proceedings of Annual Meeting* 67: 359, 1976.
42. Grabowski, H. C., Vernon, J. M., and Thomas, L. G. "The Effects of Regulatory Policy on the Incentives to Innovate: International Comparative Analysis, Presented Before the Third Seminar on Pharmaceutical Public Policy Issues." College of Public Affairs, American University, Washington, D.C., December 15, 1975.
43. Greer, A. L. *Hospital Adoption of Medical Technology: A Preliminary Investigation into Hospital Decision-Making.* Milwaukee, Wis.: The University of Wisconsin-Milwaukee, Urban Research Center, 1977.
44. Haverkamp, A. D., et al. "The Evaluation of Continuous Fetal Heart Rate Monitoring in High-Risk Pregnancy." *Am. J. Obstet. Gynecol.* 125: 310, 1976.
45. Havighurst, C. "Federal Regulation of the Health Care Delivery System: A Foreword in the Nature of a 'Package Insert.' " *University of Toledo Law Review* 6: 577, 1975.
46. Health Services Administration. *Professional Standards Review Organizations: Program Evaluation, Executive Summary.* Washington, D.C.: Department of Health, Education, and Welfare, October, 1977.
47. Hellinger, F. J. "The Effect of Certificate-of-Need Legislation on Hospital Investment." *Inquiry* XIII: 187, 1976.
48. Hiatt, H. H. "Protecting the Medical Commons: Who Is Responsible?" *N.E.J.M.* 293: 235, 1975.
49. Iglehart, J. K. "The Cost and Regulation of Medical Technology: Future Policy Directions." *MMFQ/Health and Society* 55: 25, 1977.
50. *Improving Health Care Through Research and Development, Report of the Panel on Health Services Research and Development of the President's Science Advisory Committee.* Washington, D.C.: U.S. Government Printing Office, 1972.
51. *Investigation of the National Institutes of Health.* Prepared by the Staff for the Use of the Committee on Interstate and Foreign Commerce, U.S. House of Representatives. Washington, D.C.: U.S. Government Printing Office, 1976.
52. Jonsson, E., and Marke, L. A. "Computer Assisted Tomography of the Head." Economic Analysis for Sweden, Stockholm, Sweden: *SPRI,* July 1976.
53. Kaluzny, A. D. "Innovation in Health Services, Theoretical Framework and Review of Research." *Health Serv. Res.* 9: 101, 1974.
54. Kaluzny, A. D., Veney, J. E., and Gentry, J. T. "Innovation of Health Services: A Comparative Study of Hospitals and Health Departments." *MMFQ/Health and Society* 52: 51, 1974.
55. Kaprio, L. "The Health Care Picture of Europe." In *Health Services Systems in the European Economic Community.* Hyattsville, Md.: Health Re-

sources Administration, Department of Health, Education, and Welfare, 1975, p. 10 (DHEW Publication No. HRA 76-638).

56. Klein, R. "The Rise and Decline of Policy Analysis: The Strange Case of Health Policy Making in Britain." *Policy Analysis* 2: 459, 1976.
57. Lalonde, M. *"A New Perspective on the Health of Canadians."* Ottawa, Canada: Government of Canada, 1974.
58. Lasagna, L. "Research, Regulation, and Development of New Pharmaceuticals: Past, Present and Future." *Am. J. Med. Sci.* 263: 66, 1972.
59. Lewin & Associates. *Government Controls on the Health Care System: The Canadian Experience.* Washington, D. C.: Lewin & Associates, 1976.
60. Arthur D. Little and Industrial Research Institute. *Barriers to Innovation in Industry: Opportunities for Public Policy Changes.* Washington, D.C.: Arthur D. Little, 1973 (National Science Foundation Contracts No. NSF-C748 and C725).
61. Mahler, H. Health—A Demystification of Medical Technology. *Lancet* 2: 829, 1975.
62. Mansfield, E., et al. *Research and Innovation in the Modern Corporation,* New York: W. W. Norton & Company, 1971.
63. Maxwell, R. *Health Care, the Growing Dilemma, Needs versus Resources in Western Europe, the US and the USSR.* London: McKinsey & Company, Inc. (A McKinsey Survey Report), 1975.
64. McKeown, T. "A Historical Appraisal of the Medical Task." In G. McLachlan, and T. McKeown, eds., *Medical History and Medical Care,* New York: Oxford University Press, 1971.
65. McLachlan, G. *Challenges for Change, Essays on the Next Decade in the National Health Service.* London: Oxford University Press, 1971.
66. ———. *Measuring for Management: Quantitative Methods in Health Service Management.* London: Oxford University Press, 1975.
67. ———. *Positions, Movements and Direction in Health Services Research.* London: Oxford University Press, 1974.
68. ———. ed. *A Question of Quality? Roads to Assurance in Medical Care.* London: Oxford University Press, 1976.
69. Mechanic, D. "The Growth of Medical Technology and Bureaucracy: Implications for Medical Care." *MMFQ/Health and Society* 55: 61, 1977.
70. ———. *Public Expectations and Health Care.* New York: Wiley-Interscience (John Wiley & Sons), 1972.
71. National Academy of Sciences. *Medical Technology and the Health Care System: A Study of Equipment-Embodied Technology.* Washington, D.C.: The National Research Council and the Institute of Medicine, 1978 (draft).
72. National Institutes of Health. *Inventory of Clinical Trials, Fiscal Year 1975.* Bethesda, Md.: Division of Research Grants, National Institutes of Health, 1977.
73. ———. *The Responsibilities of NIH at the Health Research/Health Care Interface.* Bethesda, Md.: Report of the Office of the Director, National Institutes of Health, February 14, 1977.
74. Neuhauser, D., and Jonsson, E. "Managerial Response to New Health Care Technology: Coronary Artery Bypass Surgery." In W. J. Abernathy, A.

Sheldon, and C. K. Prahalad, eds., *The Management of Health Care.* Cambridge, Mass.: Ballinger Publishing Co., 1974, pp. 205–213.

75. Noll, R. "The Consequences of Public Utility Regulation of Hospitals." In *Controls on Health Care.* Washington, D.C.: National Academy of Sciences, 1975, pp. 25–48.
76. *Policy Implications of the Computed Tomography (CT) Scanner.* Washington, D.C.: U.S. Government Printing Office, August 1978.
77. Office of Technology Assessment. *Development of Medical Technology: Opportunities for Assessment.* Washington, D.C.: U.S. Government Printing Office, 1976.
78. ———. *Assessing the Efficacy and Safety of Medical Technologies.* Washington, D.C.: U.S. Government Printing Office, September 1978.
79. Organisation for Economic Cooperation and Development. *Changing Priorities for Government R&D.* Paris: Organisation for Economic Cooperation and Development, 1975.
80. Paradise, J. L. "Pittsburgh Tonsillectomy and Adenoidectomy Study: Differences from Earlier Studies and Problems of Execution." *Ann. Otol. Rhinol. Laryngol.* 84: 15, 1975.
81. Peltzman, S. *Regulation of Pharmaceutical Innovation, the 1962 Amendments.* Washington, D.C.: American Enterprise Institute for Public Policy Research, 1974.
82. President's Biomedical Research Panel. *Report of the President's Biomedical Research Panel.* Washington, D.C.: U.S. Department of Health, Education, and Welfare, April 30, 1976 (DHEW Publication No. OS 76-500).
83. Preston, T. A. *Coronary Artery Surgery: A Critical Review.* New York: Raven Press, 1977.
84. Rapoport, J. *Diffusion of Technological Innovation in Hospitals: A Case Study of Nuclear Medicine.* South Hadley, Mass., 1976 (photocopy).
85. Reinhardt, U. E. *National Health Insurance in Australia, Canada, France, West Germany, and the Netherlands: A Synopsis.* Prepared for the National Center for Health Services Research International Workshop on Health Insurance, September 25–27, 1977.
86. Rettig, R. A.: *Cancer Crusade: The Story of the National Cancer Act of 1971.* Princeton, N.J.: Princeton University Press, 1977.
87. Rettig, R. A., Sorg, J. D., and Milward, H. B. *Criteria for the Allocation of Resources to Research and Development: A Review of the Literature.* Washington, D.C.: National Science Foundation, 1974.
88. Roemer, M. I. "Regulation in Different Types of Health Care Systems." In M. I. Roemer, *Health Care Systems in World Perspective.* Ann Arbor, Mich.: Health Administration Press, 1976, pp. 269–278.
89. Rogers, E. M., and Shoemaker, F. F. *Communication of Innovations, A Cross-Cultural Approach.* New York: The Free Press, 1971.
90. Rothenberg, E. *Regulation and Expansion of Health Facilities: The Certificate of Need Experience in New York State.* New York: Praeger, 1976.
91. Rothschild, Lord *A Framework for Government Research and Development.* London: Her Majesty's Stationery Office, 1971.

92. Russell, L. "The Diffusion of New Hospital Technologies in the United States." *Int. J. Health Serv.* 6: 557, 1976.
93. Russell, L. B. *Making Rational Decisions About Medical Technology.* Presented Before the American Medical Association's National Commission on the Cost of Medical Care, Chicago, Ill., November 23, 1976.
94. Salkever, D., and Bice, T. "The Impact of Certificate-of-Need Controls on Hospital Investment." *MMFQ/Health and Society* 54: 185, 1976.
95. Schifrin, L. G., and Tayan, J. R. "The Drug Lag: An Interpretive Review of the Literature." *Int. J. Health Serv.* 7: 359, 1977.
96. Schroeder, S. A., and Showstack, J. A. *The Dynamics of Medical Technology Use: Analysis and Policy Options.* Presented at the Sun Valley Forum on National Health, Sun Valley, Idaho, August 1–5, 1977.
97. Scitovsky, A. A. "Changes in Treatment and the Costs of 'Common' Illness." Presented at the Sun Valley Forum on National Health, Sun Valley, Idaho, August 1–5, 1977.
98. Sedeuilh, M. "Requirements and Data Availability for Health Care Systems in Europe." In M. F. Collen, ed., *Proceedings of an International Conference on Health Technology Systems, San Francisco.* Potomac, Md.: Health Applications Section, Operations Research Society of America, 1974, pp. 65–87.
99. Shepard, D. *Analysis of Biomedical Research, Fourth Aspect of Task, An Analysis of How New Technology is Diffused Throughout the Health Care System.* Report Prepared for the Office of Health Policy Analysis and Research, Department of Health, Education, and Welfare, August 29, 1973.
100. Sherman, H. "Research, Development and Innovation in Health Care Organizations." In W. J. Abernathy, A. Sheldon, and C. K. Prahalad, eds., *The Management of Health Care.* Cambridge, Mass.: Ballinger Publishing Co., 1974, pp. 105–124.
101. Simmons, H. E. "The Drug Regulatory System of the United States Food and Drug Administration: A Defense of Current Requirements for Safety and Efficacy." *Int. J. Health Serv.* 4: 95, 1974.
102. Spingarn, N. D. *Heartbeat: The Politics of Health Research.* Washington, D.C., Robert B. Luce, 1976.
103. Strickland, S. P. *Politics, Science, & Dread Disease,* Cambridge, Mass.: Harvard University Press, 1972.
104. Thomas, L. *Aspects of Biomedical Science Policy,* Address to the Institute of Medicine Fall Meeting. Occasional Paper of the Institute of Medicine. Washington, D.C.: National Academy of Sciences, 1972.
105. Thomas, L. *The Lives of a Cell.* New York: The Viking Press, 1974.
106. Van Langendonck, J. "Social Health Insurance in the E.E.C." In *Health Services Systems in the European Economic Community.* Hyattsville, Md.: Health Resources Administration, Department of Health, Education, and Welfare, 1975, p. 64 (DHEW Publication No. HRA 76-638).
107. "The Veterans Administration Cooperative Randomized Study of Surgery for Coronary Arterial Occlusive Disease." *Circulation* 54 (December 1976, Supp. 3).

108. "Veterans Administration Cooperative Study Group on Antihypertensive Agents." *J.A.M.A.* 202: 1028, 1967, and *J.A.M.A.* 213: 1143, 1970.
109. Wagner, J. L., and Zubkoff, M. "Medical Technology and Hospital Costs." In M. Zubkoff, I. E. Raskin, and R. S. Hanft, eds., *Hospital Cost Containment: Selected Notes for Future Policy.* New York: Prodist, 1978, p. 263.
110. Waldman, S. *The Effect of Changing Technology on Hospital Costs.* Research and Statistics Note No. 4—1972. Washington, D.C., Office of Research and Statistics, Social Security Administration, February 28, 1972.
111. Ward, G. W. *Memorandum from the National High Blood Pressure Education Program, National Institutes of Health, to the Office of Technology Assessment,* Washington, D. C., January 18, 1977.
112. Wardell, W. M. "British Usage and American Awareness of Some New Therapeutic Drugs." *Clin. Pharmacol. Ther.* 14: 1022, 1973.
113. Wardell, W. M. "Introduction of New Therapeutic Drugs in the United States and Great Britain: An International Comparison." *Clin. Pharmacol. Ther.* 14: 773, 1973.
114. Wardell, W. M. "Therapeutic Implications of the Drug Lag." *Clin. Pharmacol. Ther.* 15: 73, 1974.
115. Wardell, W. M., and Lasagna, L. *Regulation and Drug Development,* Washington, D.C.: American Enterprise Institute for Public Policy Research, 1975.
116. Warner, K. E. *The Cost of Capital-Embodied Medical Technology.* Prepared for the Committee on Technology and Health Care. National Academy of Sciences, July 1977.
117. Warner, K. E. "A 'Desperation-Reaction' Model of Medical Diffusion." *Health Serv. Res.* 10: 369, 1975.
118. Warner, K. "Treatment Decision-Making in Catastrophic Illness." *Med. Care* XV: 19, 1977.
119. Weinberg, A. M. "Criteria for Scientific Choice." *Minerva* 1: 159, 1963.
120. Weinstein, M. "Allocation of Subjects in Medical Experiments." *N.E.J.M.* 291: 1278, 1974.
121. Wennberg, J. E., and Gittelsohn, A. "Health Care Delivery in Maine Patterns of Use of Common Surgical Procedures." *J. Maine Med. Assoc.* 66: 123, 1975.
122. Wennberg, J., and Gittelsohn, A. "Small Area Variations in Health Care Delivery." *Science* 182: 1102, 1973.
123. White, K. L., and Murnaghan, J. H. "Health Care Policy Formation: Analysis, Information, and Research." *Int. J. Health Serv.* 3: 81, 1973.
124. Wiley, J. P. "What's Holding Up New Drug Development?" *FDA Consumer* 7: 21, 1973.
125. Willems, J., et al. *The Computed Tomography Scanner.* Presented at the Sun Valley Forum on National Health, Sun Valley, Idaho, August 1–5, 1977.
126. World Health Organization. *World Health Statistics Annual, Volume III, Health Personnel and Hospital Establishments.* Geneva: World Health Organization, 1977.

Chapter 6

Technological Innovation: Cause or Effect of Increasing Expenditures for Health?

Jean François Lacronique and Simone Sandier

SUMMARY

Innovation is becoming an increasingly important factor in the health-care area, and it is contributing to the expansion in both the quantity and the quality of medical activity.

The factors promoting this expansion are of two kinds:

1. endogenous, innovative factors that are encouraged by the investment of capital and the interpenetration of the sciences;
2. exogenous and manifold factors of a predominantly cultural and economic nature.

The consequences of this development in medical, economic, social, administrative, and industrial terms are many and varied and are the underlying reasons for the wide range of attitudes typifying what are often conflicting interests.

1. TECHNICAL INNOVATION–CAUSE OR EFFECT OF INCREASES IN HEALTH EXPENDITURES?

It is not easy to explain the marked statistical correlation between increases in consumption (and in cost) and technological progress.

There are two ways of interpreting this correlation: Innovation can be regarded either as the factor stimulating consumption or as its consequence. These two interpretations have vastly different political implications, in particular regarding the possible need to control innovation.

2. THE JUSTIFICATION FOR TECHNOLOGICAL PROGRESS

2.1. Technological Progress and the Quality of Medical Care

The prime objective of technological progress in the health field is to improve the quality of medical care. It is difficult to make an accurate assessment of the overall effect of medical care. However, effect can be broken down into its principal aspects, each of which is measurable in objective terms:

effectiveness;
safety;
economy;
convenience;
accessibility.

All these aspects are to be found at the root of progress, the scope of which goes beyond the strict limits of a mere improvement in technical efficiency; all constitute incentives to increased consumption of medical care.

2.2. Additional and Substitute Technologies

In most cases an innovation is simply incorporated as an additional weapon into the arsenal of medical treatment, except in cases when there is a total overlap of function and there is evidence of some degree of substitution.

3. THE EXTERNAL EFFECTS

The participation of and the responses made by some of those involved in the health-care system bring external effects to bear on the spread of progress.

3.1. *Researchers* in France constitute a professional body: From an international viewpoint, there are few parallels to their career patterns and their reluctance to contract with industry or develop their own inventions. What is more, they are unmistakably influenced by the English-speaking countries.

3.2. *Manufacturers* also suffer the consequences of this situation. Although the domestic market in France is growing rapidly, French manufacturers are benefiting little from this expansion.

3.3. *Physicians* are, of course, both producers and consumers of innovation. During the last ten years, there has been a substantial shift of emphasis in favor of state hospitals because of the capital investment required for purchasing new equipment.

3.4. *The public* is aware of this uneven distribution of equipment and is demanding that all should be aligned on the level of the best equipped sectors.

3.5. The *financing organizations that provide the funds* and are responsible for covering the real costs of innovation are worried by this growth. They resist it by means of structural standards (e.g., a medical services map) that are effective for a certain period of time (at the expense, however, of serious consequences in the industrial area). Their scope of action upstream (i.e., the control of the innovation or its consequences) and downstream (i.e., the control of its utilization) is relatively limited, sometimes creating a conflict of interests in which each group tends to use arguments of an emotional kind in support of its own case.

In conclusion, it should be emphasized that the problem of technical innovation in the medical area is primarily dependent on international factors (with respect to know-how as well as the exchange of ideas and information). The problem cannot be solved by isolated measures undertaken on a national scale.

The pressure that innovation exerts on the demand for and on the consumption of medical care is unavoidable and is moreover justified by the social and cultural context in which health care is dispensed. It is part of the natural logic of trends that by partially eliminating price as a factor controlling the market, the subsidizing of medicine by the state will result in control mechanisms not only at the investment level but also at the level of technical and economic evaluation.

One of the characteristic features of the medical profession's outlook is its interest in all things new, for example, the end of one's medical studies is marked by the submission of a thesis or a dissertation that, by definition, constitutes an original contribution to the store of knowledge within the young doctor's profession. This factor, like many others, has contributed to the continued extension of the scope of medical activity from both a qualitative as well as a quantitative point of view.

This process has been gaining momentum for almost thirty years. It affects every aspect of health care, for example, the areas of preventive medicine, epidemiology, vaccinations, and contraception have had a profound impact on physicians' attitudes and behavior. In the area of diagnosis, there was the introduction of various methods of laboratory estimation and pictorial recording as well as functional investigations. As far as therapy is concerned, almost all drugs, prostheses, and apparatuses supplementing vital functions currently in use are less than thirty years old.

* * *

The factors contributing to this expansion are of two kinds: First, *innovative factors,* or factors that make innovation possible, that is:

the development of research capabilities and resources;
the interpenetration of the sciences (among various branches of medicine or via contributions from other sciences, e.g., chemistry, physics, automation, etc.).

Second, *development factors* that enable innovation to be exploited and made widely available, that is:

increasing numbers in the medical profession;
modern, predominantly scientific, education;
increases in the international exchange of ideas and technologies;
improvements in the general standard of living;
the collective assumption of health charges by the systems of health insurance.

The ways in which different groups involved in the health-care system react to various incentives depend on what interests motivate them, for example, in some cases, scientific, medical, and professional interests, and, in other cases, social, economic, and administrative interests. Even attitudes toward the value of technological progress often reflect differing viewpoints.

4. TECHNICAL INNOVATION– CAUSES OR EFFECT OF INCREASES IN HEALTH EXPENDITURES?

To a large extent technological innovations are statistically closely linked to increases in health-care consumption and thereby to costs. An analysis of the various aspects of medical treatment reveals that the most rapidly increasing areas of consumption are those in which technical innovations have been the most numerous in recent years. For example, ambulatory care, laboratory analyses, and radiology have shown rapid increases, with average annual growth rates of 12.2 percent and 7.6 percent in volume, whereas traditional acts, such as home visits and GP consultations, show only slight increases—1.7 percent and 4.2 percent. (See Figure 6.1.)

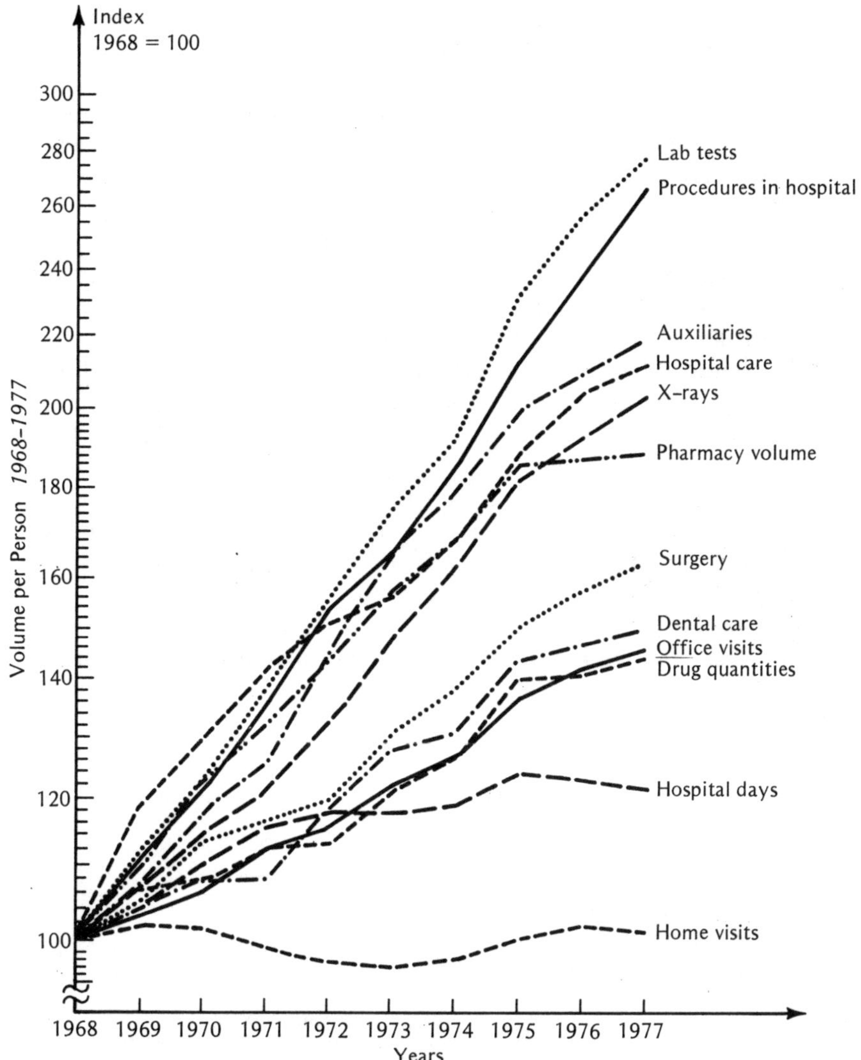

Figure 6.1. Growth in the volume of medical care, by type of care.

This trend is most marked in the case of state hospitals because hospitals are prime locations for concentrating the most advanced therapeutic techniques. The increasing proportion of hospital activity devoted to the provision of technical services is illustrated by increases in the number of radiological acts (Z) and laboratory analyses (B) per inpatient in every category of hospital. (See Table 6.1.)

Such technical acts account for an increasing share of hospital activity, as is illustrated in Figure 6.2. The effect of innovation is also evident in the area of private medicine, for example, in France in 1959, radiology accounted for 12.6 percent of private practitioners' activity; by 1976, the figure had risen to 20.2 percent.

In broad terms, technological progress, as reflected in an increased consumption of "technological" acts, accounted for about two-thirds of the increased volume of medical acts irrespective of any change in price. (See Figure 6.2.)

It is difficult to analyze the relationship between the increased pace of technological progress and the growth in expenditure in terms of cause and effect. Although technological progress would certainly seem to be the cause of the increase in the volume of medical care, its effect on costs is more complex because in a certain number of cases, one can observe that reductions in unit costs coincide with an increase in aggregate costs. The nature of this relationship is, however, of fundamental importance in defining a health policy.

If one accepts the hypothesis that the primary effect of innovation is to encourage consumption, then any attempt at improving the productivity of the health-care system should be concerned with controlling the value of an innovation during its earliest stages of development.

The alternative hypothesis suggests that technological innovation is the response of human inventiveness to legitimate needs, in which case,

Table 6.1. State General Hospitals (France)

	Number of "Zs"		*Number of "Bs"*	
	Per Inpatient	*Per Day*	*Per Inpatient*	*Per Day*
1965	22.48	1.0	153	7.3
1970	30.59	1.7	298	16.4
1973	37.54	2.4	394	25.1
	Average Annual Growth Rate (%)			
1965–1973	6.6	11.6	12.6	16.7
1970–1973	7.1	12.2	9.8	15.2

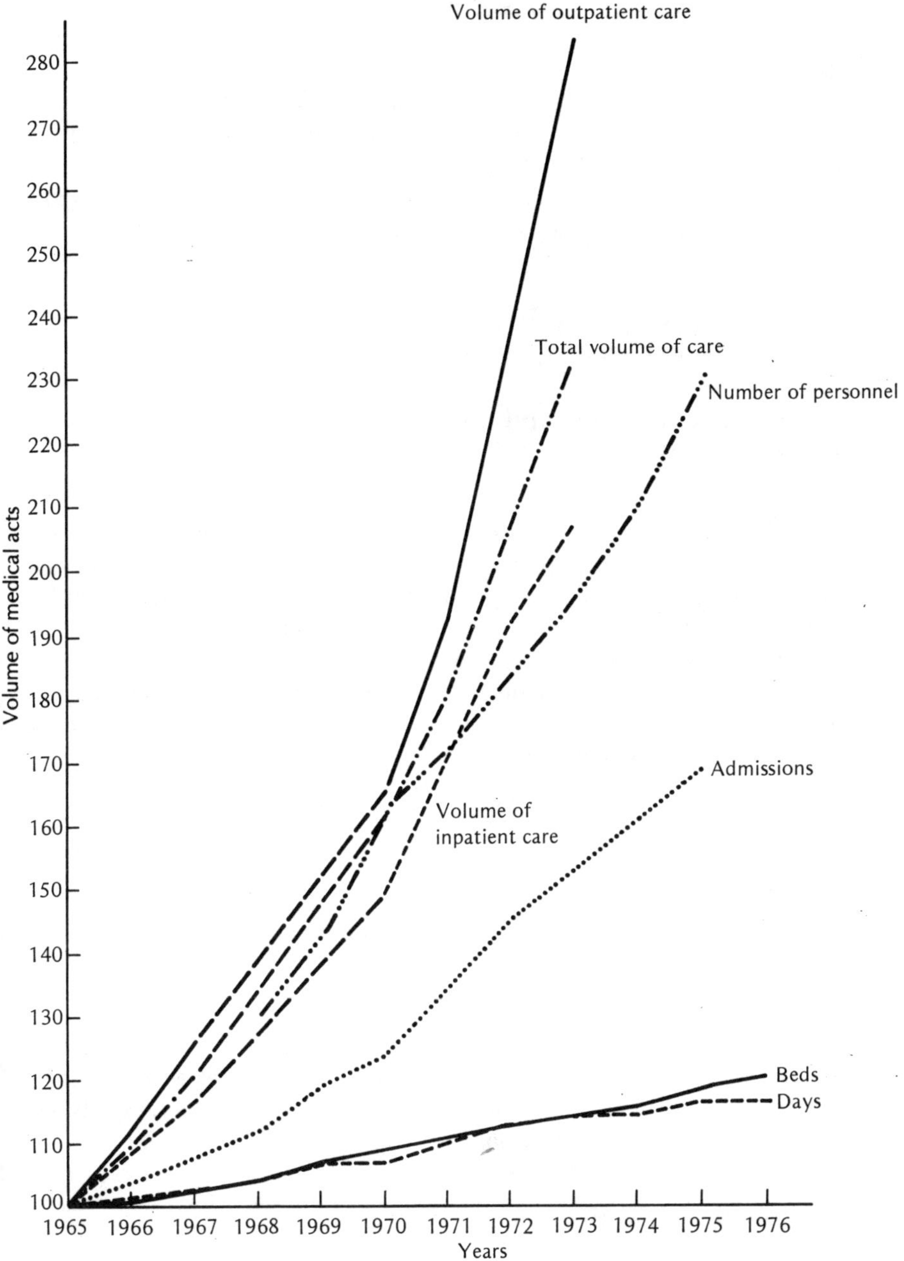

Figure 6.2. Production in hospitals.

such control should only be exercised with respect to excessive use or consumption in quantitative terms on the basis of results compiled over a period of time.

These two hypotheses are not mutually exclusive, but they differ in the degree of importance attached to their determinants. In isolated situations, they provide conflicting evidence, implying different recommendations with respect to health policy, depending on the predominance of factors favoring one or the other hypothesis.

THE JUSTIFICATION FOR TECHNOLOGICAL PROGRESS

Technological Progress and the Quality of Medical Care

As a rule, the introduction of a technological innovation is justified on the grounds of a continuing desire to improve the quality of the service provided by the health-care system. Although one generally tends to draw a distinction between the concept of qualitative (i.e., subjective) evaluation and quantitative (i.e., objective) evaluation, it is possible to assess the marginal benefit deriving from a technological advance by breaking down this concept of quality into five basic components, which are measurable in objective terms:

technical effectiveness (e.g., improved diagnosis, more effective treatment);
safety;
economy;
convenience (e.g., respect for the patient, the rapidity and the harmlessness of the treatment, etc.);
accessibility (physical and mental).

Different scales are used for the measurement of these five aspects, but the aggregate assessment of an innovation can be regarded as a "complex growth function" of the five independent variables that can be analyzed separately at first and then globally.

Technological Effectiveness

Whenever therapy is concerned, effectiveness can be measured, for example, by reductions in mortality, morbidity, and disabilities. Among the most remarkable technological advances made in the last ten years, one can mention:

- progress in chemotherapy of malignant blood diseases, which has transformed what was a fatal disease ten years ago into what is now in most cases a curable disease;
- articular prostheses (for the hip in particular), which have transformed rheumatic or traumatological pathology for the elderly;
- haemodialysis machines and transplants, which enable patients with renal failure to survive;
- intensive care, which enables many of the affected vital functions to be replaced, generating such success that it has even aroused some criticism of its possible abuse ("therapeutic overkill").

In the area of diagnosis, effectiveness is evidenced by the accuracy and specificity of investigations.

It should be mentioned in this context that scientific methods for evaluating new forms of therapy are generally applicable only to new kinds of drug and not to new kinds of equipment. Generally, several reasons are given:

- controlled therapeutic trials are necessary in the case of drugs because the expected improvements are sometimes difficult to assess, that is, purely subjective reactions are involved, and external influences need to be isolated (e.g., placebos, side effects, etc.);
- it would be impossible to use controlled therapeutic trials in the case of equipment because of the difficulty of sampling or setting up control groups;
- progress in the area of equipment is considered more tangible than progress in therapy and thus does not require the use of experimental procedures.

Economy

Certain innovations result in reductions in the unit costs of treatment.

The automation of numerous laboratory analysis techniques is a case in point, as is the development of simple tests or apparatuses (e.g., reagent paper, enzymological techniques, etc.).

It should be mentioned that the replacement of a technique by a new one is a progressive process, with the result that sometimes, at least for a time, an innovation will show a financial return when the rates of reimbursement are based on the higher cost of the previous technique.

In the case of laboratory apparatus, reductions in unit costs have contributed to the rapid spread of innovation. Ease of use and lower unit costs as a result of automation encourage a greater degree of use and may entail a rapid growth in consumption within this sector.

In addition, mention should be made of the spread of renal dialysis performed at home, its major advantage being a 50 percent reduction in the cost of treatment (and equal effectiveness, to say nothing of the psychological advantages, e.g., easier social readjustment, etc.).

Safety and Convenience

An innovation may be aimed at minimizing the risks and inconvenience that the process of treatment may involve for the patient and his or her entourage, for example:

therapeutic complications;
pain;
delay;
injuring the person's feelings, invasion of privacy;
disruption of the person's social or family life.

Increased efforts currently devoted to "noninvasive" techniques illustrate the extent to which an objective of this kind emphasizes the technical effectiveness of treatment. The following innovations are cases in point:

electrocardiography;
isotope scintillation scan;
echotomography and echocardiography (ultrasound);
thermography;
scanner.

Research in a similar direction is being carried out with a view to perfecting techniques based on magnetism (rheography), nuclear magnetic resonance (zeugmatography), stable isotopes, and so on.

The one feature that all these examinations have in common is their relative harmlessness. They can therefore be repeated without risk, and often they are based on automated techniques that make them easy to use.

Safety and automation are particularly attractive because they obviate one of the traditional limiting factors affecting the spread of technological innovation: the problem of training staff.

The obvious result is the very rapid broadening of the fields in which these techniques can be applied, the scanner being a particularly good example.

Another example is the fairly widespread use of thermography, now generally regarded as being of little diagnostic value (except for confirming a diagnosis of polycystic mastopathy of the breast, which can, however, be diagnosed histologically).

Accessibility

This last aspect is illustrated in France by such organizational innovations as "home hospitalization" and "day hospitals." These innovations facilitate access to health care of a high quality without resorting to the traditional system of hospitalization. In the future, improvements in telecommunications service (teleprocessing, better organization of hospital appointments, long-distance consultations, etc.) will tend to promote easier access to the health-care system. The outcome will inevitably be an increase in demand. Unless a substitution effect can be achieved through a reduction in the intake capacity of existing health-care facilities, one can expect that these innovations will result in a corresponding increase in consumption through the addition of telecommunications services to existing services.

By and large, any improvement involving one of the five variables, even when improvement does not affect the system's technical efficiency, can be considered a contribution to the quality of health care.

In certain cases one could envisage an improved overall result, even if an innovation were to dilute one of the variables, provided that this impact was offset by an increase in the results of one or more of the other variables. For example, certain therapies to reduce pain in cases of terminal cancer sometimes provide greater degrees of relief at the price of shortening patients' lives. On the other hand, one sometimes prefers to take the added risk of a difficult operation in the hope that it will prove effective.

If one accepts this line of argument and the premise that substitutions occur in the "quality of health care," one can then borrow one of the classic equations used in the economics of market goods and services and construct a "demand function" in which the "price" variable (variations that affect consumption) would successively be replaced by the variables "risk," "pain" (or inconvenience), and "difficulty of access." Intuitively one assumes that any improvement in these factors is likely to stimulate demand. Empirical observations that provide evidence of an increased consumption of technical medical acts reflect this logical and legitimate trend.

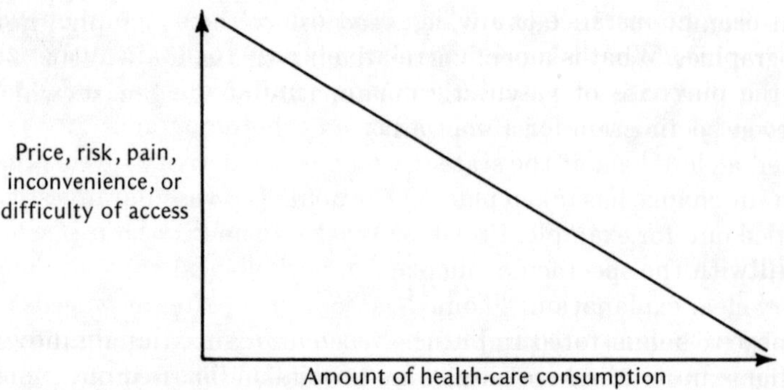

Addition and Substitution of Technologies

The spread of every new technology does not, of course, follow the same pattern. In some cases the new technology is effective—simple to apply and inexpensive. There is therefore no obstacle to its rapid spread, which in fact sometimes takes place. Usually, however, new technology is complex; its application requires the purchase of equipment and the training of medical personnel; it is expensive; and in many cases its effectiveness cannot be measured at the time it is introduced but only after studies conducted over a period of years have been analyzed.

For these reasons, innovations in methods of diagnosis or therapy will more often than not be included as *additional elements* in the health-care process. From the point of view of the economics of the operation, cost will in most cases be ignored or inadequately assessed, and only the results from the health-care point of view will be taken into account: However unimportant these results prove to be, they will nonetheless be subjected to thorough analysis (i.e., theses, dissertations, reports, demonstrations, etc.) because each principal involved in the health-care system will ascribe values different from those that would result from a simple interplay of market forces.

The most striking example of a technology adopted as an addition to existing techniques is provided by the recent development in radiological techniques for vascular investigation: Angiography, a technique that has been in use for several decades, is expensive, risky, and painful.

The necessary equipment is very expensive (approximately half a million Francs), and in France the official formula was one unit for every million inhabitants. One might have expected that with the development of the scanner and echotomography around 1975, the situation would have been reversed because these two techniques reduce the need for vascular radiography. However, since these two techniques became available, the activity of vascular radiology departments has not declined.

There has been no instance of any significant decrease in the frequency of arteriographies. What is more, it is relatively easy to obtain authorization for the purchase of vascular radiology units, whereas it is very difficult to get permission for a scanner or an echotomograph.

However, a close look at the statistics on medical activity reveals that an important change has taken place in the quality of vascular investigations carried out, for example, Professor Wackenheim (Strasburg), when confronted with the spectacular increase in pathological angiographies, gave a very clear explanation: "Tomodensitometry creates new needs for angiography (to define, for example, the vascular origin of lesions discovered by the scanner), and investigations of this kind carried out by radiology departments have replaced certain angiographies which are no longer necessary."

Genuine substitutions, however, sometimes occur, for example:

direct estimations have replaced the investigation of numerous functions (thyroid, adrenal, pituitary, gonads);
in surgery, prostheses have eliminated the earlier kinds of appliances;
in drug therapy, one antibiotic will be superseded by another (*Rifampicin* has replaced *Rimifon* and *PAS*);
in preventive medicine, vaccinations have rendered certain equipment unnecessary (sanatoria, respiratory reeducation for poliomyelitis victims). For a technology to be treated as a substitute, it must supersede the previous technique. If not, there is a good chance that it will simply be added to the existing series of medical acts, thereby raising the problem of its marginal benefit in relation to its cost.

External Effects

In addition to the direct effects of innovation on the process of medical care, there are indirect or external effects that stem from the participation of and the responses to innovation made by different sectors of the health-care system.

Researchers. At the origin of every innovation is the activity of research laboratories working not only in the areas of medicine and biology but also in sciences that seem, a priori, remote from the medical sector, for example, physics, chemistry, automation, and so on. The present tendency is to seek acknowledgment of success in the research field primarily through recognition by fellow research workers (i.e., published works, symposia, internal promotion) and to ignore the industrial, social, and economic implications of the results of one's research.

One should stress the international character of the dissemination of knowledge in this field through the agency of international publications and symposia that gives considerable weight to the "Anglo-Saxon" influence that constitutes an undeniable cultural and linguistic handicap for the French. This international context means that the emergence of innovations is governed only to a limited extent by a country's research policy. Thus whereas a policy of austerity in the context of an unfavorable economic climate (particularly in a country where research is institutionalized) may well result in a decline in the productivity of that country's research workers in terms of inventions, innovations will nonetheless continue to be made in other countries and will sustain demand at the consumer level.

It is feared, however, that the consumers' remoteness from the source of innovation makes more difficult the assimilation (and therefore the improvement) as well as the use of such imported technology. Therefore, it may well be the case that for certain research teams, innovation consists of relabeling or even of transferring foreign inventions to France. There are numerous examples, the scanner being the most recent.

Manufacturers. The biomedical-technology sector of industry is expanding rapidly: Although there has been a falling off in the growth rates for pharmaceutical products on the domestic market in terms of volume and turnover (respectively, +2% and +9.9% in 1976), the export market showed a growth of 20 percent in the same year.

In the biomedical-equipment sector, where international competition is increasing rapidly, the value of the French domestic market expanded at an average rate of 13.3 percent per year between 1971 and 1976. This growth rate is one of the highest in the world—exceeded only by Japan and Germany. Paradoxically, the growth rate of the American domestic market is only approximately 8 percent, despite the fact that the United States devotes by far the greatest efforts of any country in the world to research and development.

Roughly half the turnover in this area is accounted for by the purchase of equipment for radiology and nuclear medicine, the only sector in which French industry can claim to be of some importance at the international level.

Despite considerable efforts to encourage applied research (joint-venture agreements, the pooling of resources, development grants, etc.), the French biomedical-equipment industry has been unable to mount an effective counteroffensive on the international market, and the growth of its domestic market has in fact benefited foreign importers to a far greater extent than French manufacturers, as illustrated in Table 6.2 that shows growth in the market share for foreign imports for 1969–1971.

Table 6.2. Evolution of the Market for Biomedical Equipment in France

Imports	*1969*	*1970*	*1971*
United States	7.03%	9.08%	10.66%
Germany	16.84%	17.53%	21.61%
United Kingdom	2.79%	3.93%	5.30%
The Netherlands	3.69%	3.64%	5.15%
Italy	3.08%	3.86%	4.81%
Others	9.39%	12.62%	17.50%
Total Share of French Market	42.80%	50.66%	63.03%

Source: French Foreign Trade Statistics

There is virtually no domestic production of laboratory apparatus in France (with the exception of an automatic sample analyzer for isotope studies) or fiber-optic endoscopes, extracorporeal-circulation and respiratory-assistance machines, haematological or endocrinological analyzers, scintillation cameras, and so on.

Some success, however, has been achieved in the areas of renal dialysis, pictorial recording in nuclear medicine, and ultrasound. In every instance, success involved initial discoveries by university research units, which are encouraged by the government to enter into some form of contractual agreement or joint venture with manufacturers. In most cases, the major obstacle confronting those who attempt to arrange these "marriages" is the considerable difference between the two partners in terms of motivation, which is accentuated by the disparity between the funds allotted to the research team and to the manufacturer. What is more, there is never any a posteriori assessment of these joint ventures. The lack of assessment tends to encourage misconceptions or sharp practices that are confined to areas so highly specialized and restricted that they manage to escape public attention. In the final analysis, despite the vast sums allocated to research and development and the interesting areas for innovation proposed by some French laboratories, one is obliged to acknowledge the limited contribution made by France to the development of instrument technology over the past fifteen years. One should mention, however, the periodic improvements in existing technologies, such as the atomic pacemaker and the Rhône-Poulenc dialysis membrane.

This critical analysis may suggest an attack aimed at the structures and the way programs are administered in research organizations and industry in France. In fact, although the examples of certain foreign countries like Germany or Sweden are evidence of the fact that it is possible to achieve industrial success on a European scale, it would seem that the fundamental problem lies in the disparity between the effort that the United States devotes to this area and what is possible in other countries. As one of the persons in charge of the development of dialyzers at Rhône-Poulenc maintains, the biomedical-equipment industry can no longer limit itself to a national or even a regional market. The market has become worldwide, and any set of rules has to acknowledge this fact; purely national regulation, as in the case of the scanner in France, runs the risk of being ignored and of creating consequences far more serious than those it was designed to avoid.

Physicians. Physicians, in particular those whose activities are covered by the 1964 hospital reform that instituted the threefold function of "teaching/treatment/research," are both producers and consumers of innovations. They are stimulated in this respect by their awareness of the imperfections of their diagnostic and therapeutic techniques and their desire to provide better treatment. They are influenced by a powerful network of medical information: France has two daily papers entirely devoted to medical news and almost three hundred specialist publications.

They are sometimes motivated by the promotional efforts of manufacturers attempting to develop specific markets (e.g., for haemodialysis machines, scanners, ultraviolet chambers or "puvatherapy," fiber-optic endoscopes, etc.), but basic costs of recent technological innovations tend to put them out of the reach of small, privately-financed medical teams. This reason explains the distortion that has occurred over the past three years in the structure of the market for radiological apparatus in France—a distortion that has conduced to the benefit of state institutions and to the detriment of the private sector.

The Public. The attitude of the general public remains one of the determining factors because it is particularly sensitive to arguments relating to effectiveness, convenience, and safety. The public as a whole acknowledges as unfair disparities in terms of equipment and access to health care, and the technical nature of the problem is almost always understood as a guarantee of quality. Those responsible for providing medical care are aware of this attitude and therefore seek to satisfy the continuing demand for technological progress. This kind of demand, for instance, is one reason why scanners have "taken off" in the United States—a case of "keeping up with the Joneses."

Several factors have been at work in this area, for example, one of the most important developments affecting the health-care area in France has been the progressive extension of health insurance to cover every member of the population. This extension represents a major social achievement aimed at reducing the inequalities of access to good quality medical care, such inequalities being considered primarily the result of differences in personal income. This development has ensured that the cost of increasingly complex medical technology no longer constitutes an acceptable form of social discrimination.

Allowing every patient access to the same kind of medical care has caused an increase in demand. It should be mentioned that this social reform coincided with a period of extraordinary industrial and technological progress. As a result, early diagnosis has increased the awareness of apparent morbidity and thereby created a demand for health care; generally, technological progress inevitably leads to an increase in "conscious needs," to requirements governing the quality of the results obtained, and to a reduced number of errors, omissions, and failures. Thus whereas inequalities are increasingly regarded as unacceptable, they are becoming more frequent. For instance, because the spread of new equipment is not an instantaneous process, certain consumers will have access to it before others. There is also evidence of wide disparities in consumption among socioprofessional categories and regions.

In the area of radiology, the figures show that in France the rural population's consumption is fifty percent below the national average and that the variations among "departments" (administrative districts, of which there are one hundred in France) range from one to five; moreover, it is apparent that more backward regions do not succeed in catching up with the leaders over the course of time.

Financing Organizations. Health-insurance organizations have the dual responsibility of providing equitable access to health care and necessary funds. These two factors condition their attitudes toward technological innovation. The question that they ask themselves is, Which innovations appear to be valid and therefore merit widespread adoption, and which are of a more questionable value? Their aim is to control decisions regarding initial investments that are often substantial, entail considerable overhead costs, and have to be amortized in the scale of reimbursements for examinations and treatment.

In France therefore there is a "medical-services map" designed to limit the number of expensive pieces of equipment. These regulations make it mandatory for all those wishing to acquire "expensive equipment," that is, equipment costing more than F.F.100,000, to submit their requests to a ministerial committee responsible for ensuring that guidelines are respected. These regulations apply equally to the public as well as to the private sector. According to these guidelines, "requirements" for scanners, for example, should not exceed one unit for every million inhabitants, echotomographs (ultrasound) one unit for every five hundred thousand inhabitants, and so on.

Needless to say, these norms are arbitrary and are formulated by the committee on the basis of criteria of very unequal weight. In most cases, the sole purpose of these norms is to be restrictive and prevent the chaotic proliferation of equipment.

From this point of view, the new law has proved very effective. For example, the first scanner was not installed in France until 1975, by which time its neighbors had acquired several machines. By April 1978, there were 22 machines in operation (14 head and 8 whole body), compared with 30 in the Netherlands, 28 in England, and 200 in Japan.

When one questions social security officials, they willingly admit to being the prime opponents within the administration of the spread of new technology. In their view, any innovation, however efficient, involves the risk of increased consumption without necesssarily guaranteeing better results in terms of patients' health.

In every country, government officials, at least as much as the medical profession, have been responsible for requiring "evaluations of technologies," whereas, until recently, physicians' expertise was regarded as sufficient. In the area of treatment, for instance, medical judgment used to be a sufficiently valid criterion for authorizing the introduction of a drug. No form of regulation regarding the nature and the length of its trial period had been required.

CONCLUSIONS

The international character of problems relating to innovation in the health-care area affects the various stages of its introduction and adoption.

Because of the international impact of scientific publications and exchanges, research activity in any one country can influence the introduction of an innovation throughout the world. Industry's markets stretch well beyond national borders, and marketing policies embrace many countries. Those responsible for a nation's health policy have to pay heed to pressures exerted by consumers of medical care in the context of international rivalry. National policies therefore have only limited effects on the development and adoption of innovations that seem to have become inescapable phenomena in developing economies.

Innovations in health care have brought about progress in the areas of prevention, diagnosis, and therapy. But innovation does not solve two problems related to the consumption of health care:

First, because the widespread introduction of any innovation takes time, this lag tends to arouse awareness of the inequalities of access to health care.

Second, in most cases, innovation tends to create a demand for health care, causing an increase in health expenditure even when it reduces the unit costs of certain treatments or diagnoses.

By raising the problem of setting limits to the spread of innovations, these factors invariably provide incentives to financing organizations to set up control procedures directed toward assessing economic, social, and technological justifications for change.

Chapter 7

Technology in Medical Diagnosis: Aspects of Its Dynamic and Impact

Stuart S. Blume

I. PERSPECTIVES ON THE PROBLEM

The technological component of health care is an issue likely to receive increasing attention in the near future. Growing government concern, notably, in the United States, is a function partly of the identification of technological and technical change as important contributants to rising health-care (and especially hospital) costs.[1] Whereas process innovation in industry is commonly directed at cost reduction, this objective seems almost never to be the case in the health system (Iglehart, 1977). Moreover, the benefits in terms of improved health (especially when this result is considered in cost-benefit terms) are often uncertain or disputed, even by some in the medical profession.

Resulting government concern is likely to be expressed in the form of necessary evaluations (as is commonly the case with drugs prior to licensing), attempts at regulation (as in American certificate-of-need rulings (Bice; Banta) and French norms (Kervasdoué). In the United Kingdom, where the concentration of hospital facilities in the National Health Service and concomitant state financing would seem to make control relatively simple, concern has recently been expressed at the lack of information about equipment used in and bought for the health service as well as the lack of procedures to evaluate medical equipment (DHSS, 1978).

It is evident that the rapidity with which new technologies diffuse through the medical system is the most immediate cause of technology-derived cost inflation. Although this problem is not the one to which this chapter is principally addressed (for reasons that will be outlined below), some points should be made.

A. Diffusion of Medical Technologies: Technical Change

It seems clear that the process of innovation in medical technology can be understood in much the same way as the diffusion of innovations is generally explained. For example, Russell has recently shown how the familiar "S" curve is obtained in plotting the diffusion through the American hospital system of a wide array of new technologies, ranging from intensive-care units through radio-therapy facilities to renal-dialysis units (1976). Nevertheless, although it is possible to generalize about diffusion processes in a wide range of innovating communities, specifics are also important. Groups and communities differ in their propensities to innovate, inclinations that derive from differences in values, norms, and goals. The process of technical change in medicine cannot be understood in terms of generalizations alone but must take account the unique nature of medicine as a set of values, as knowledge, and as a system of social action.

Much social-scientific writing on health matters is concerned with elucidating these factors, the effects of medical values, and the cognitive framework of medicine from a distinct perspective. Although social scientists necessarily have their own disciplinary frameworks for understanding change in medicine, the terms in which practitioners debate, for example, the relative merits of alternative available technologies, must also be important to analysts. Such debate offers a crucial insight into the values, commitments, and priorities of the profession vis-à-vis technology.

Most social scientists agree on the commitment of the medical profession to maximum technological sophistication. Fuchs (1968), for example, argues, "The physician's approach to medical care and health is dominated by what may be called a 'technologic imperative.' In other words, medical tradition emphasizes giving the best care that is technically possible; the only legitimate and explicitly recognized constraint is the state of the art."

Insofar as this approach is operational, such commitments differentiate the medical profession from many communities in which the diffusion of innovation may be studied. There are other specifics that must be recognized as important to the diffusion process. One is the way in which the availability of a new technology stimulates the discovery of many applications far beyond that for which it was originally designed.

Ultrasonic scanning, discussed below, is a case in point. It has been used since the early 1960s in obstetrics. In recent years, however, its use has spread to such diverse fields as neurology, ophthalmology, cardiology, and the detection of tumors in such organs as the kidney, liver, prostate, and uterus. Russell reported a similar spread in the application of so different a technology as the intensive-care unit (1976). It should not be necessary to state that the effects, the value, and the cost benefits will not necessarily be the same in new areas of application as in the original ones. For example, it may well be, as Russell suggested, that although intensive care offers benefits—in the form of reduced mortality rates—to those with myocardial infarction, there is no evidence of its value elsewhere, despite average costs three to five times higher than those incurred in caring for a patient on a normal ward.

A further way in which the diffusion of new medical technologies can be stimulated is through the pressure of public opinion, often mediated by political action. Health is often perceived as a fundamental value in Western society, and it seems likely that the medical identification of "best practice" with "newest technology" has its place in popular beliefs. The news media can create demand. In the United Kingdom, for example, a debate is taking place over the desirability of a nationwide screening program for certain foetal defects. (More is said below about the tests involved.) Medical interests are divided on the desirability of such a procedure. Nevertheless, a newspaper with a wide circulation carried an article that began: "Britain is rapidly coming nearer to the day when EVERY expectant mother can fulfil her dearest wish—that the child she is carrying will be born normal."

B. Technological Change

Because this diffusion process and the resulting overprovision of expensive facilities most clearly show the relation between innovation and rising costs, it is an obvious focus for government regulation. But because it amounts to the attempt to control a process legitimated by values very close to the heart of the medical profession, regulation will necessarily encounter substantial resistance. Moreover, because it will appear to be a struggle over the extent to which "best possible treatment" should be made available, there is every expectation of public support for doctors. The facts of consumer choice in the (still relatively) free-market system of the United States show that this attitude has hitherto prevailed.

Hence a case can be made for early intervention in the process by which new techniques become available. Technology assessment—the evaluation of the direct and the indirect costs and benefits of new devices before they are made available commercially—could be an important aspect of this process (OTA, 1976; Banta). Evaluation is certainly implicit in the view that not only costs but the effectiveness and safety of new modes of diagnosis or therapy are important concerns of government. Technology assessment, insofar as it has been developed, focuses on individual (discrete) existing technologies. Little attention has been devoted to understanding the process of technological change at preceding stages of development.

There is, however, a substantial literature on the process of technological change, although almost none of it deals with medical innovation. Many of these studies are economic in scope, and economists can turn to some twenty years of accumulating empirical work on innovation and technology.

Much of the early work was concerned with estimating the contribution of technical change to economic growth or productivity increases at the national level by ascertaining what was unexplained by known increases in capital and labor inputs. More recently, much interest has developed in understanding the determinants of successful innovation at the level of the firm or industrial sector (Freeman, 1977). "Successful Innovation," in such studies, is defined in commercial, not technical, terms, that is, in terms of the profit accruing to the innovating firm. Economists can quite properly argue, for example, that aerospace R&D has made too little a contribution to the British economy because the industry judges success purely in terms of technical criteria relating to effective performance. Some economists have attempted to measure the return on innovation not to the innovating firm but to society. Griliches, for example, studied the rate of return on American investment in research on hybrid seed corn. He found that although the benefit to society had been very large, the commercial interests involved had not taken advantage of this development: "Almost none of the calculated social returns from hybrid corn were appropriated by the hybrid seed industry or by corn producers. They were passed on to consumers in the form of lower prices and higher output." (1958). This work, like most recent work on the economics of technological innovation, focused on *specific* innovations (or associated inventions).

One economist who focused on *classes* of inventions was Schmookler. After considering patent data over long periods, he concluded that historical shifts in the extent of inventive activity in given sectors of the economy (e.g., petroleum refining and railroads) followed shifts in the output of those sectors. In other words, Schmookler's view was that the rate of technological change, or the extent of inventive activity, in a given sector is principally determined by the level of economic activity in that sector (1966). Although it does not deal with the nature or the direction of change, Schmookler's work amounts to a (partial) theory of technological change rather than of economic growth.

Some, not all, of this "inventive activity" amounts to the assimilation of the results of research in new products or processes. In the medical area, indeed, the growth of government funding of biomedical R&D has been based on the assumption that such research will lead to new methods of treatment or cure. In the United Kingdom, policy in the past few years has prescribed relating the performance of biomedical research to identified medical (rather than purely scientific) priorities. Hence the curious paradox to which Iglehart (1977) has drawn attention: Governments have increasingly funded R&D designed to produce modes of treatment that then place increasing burdens on health-care budgets!

There is also a second strand to the problem. It has been suggested that a constraint on the expansion of inventive activity in industry (i.e., within firms producing medical equipment, often of a sophisticated electronic kind) has been the small size of the market (relative to other markets open to firms engaged in electronic R&D) and hence profits. But this situation may be changing, as the example of the CAT scanner indicates. In other words, it is possible that economic incentives to increase industrial invention could also be growing, especially bearing in mind the multinational markets available.

Thus at a time of increasing government concern with technological contributions to health costs, both economic forces and emphasis on biomedical R&D could stimulate an increase in the rate of technological change.

Hence a proper understanding of the *dynamics* of technological change (the forces that serve to determine both the rate and the direction of such change) in medicine is essential to any attempt at planning in the health area.

Planning must reflect a better understanding of the response of the medical profession to technological change (which is not, it must be understood, generally on the scale of the CAT scanner). In other words, what is needed is an approach that views technological change as a continuous process, with its own rate and direction, rather than simply as the successive appearance of a few wholly novel devices.

The focus of this paper is more limited. As a partial attempt at understanding the dynamics and the nature of change, it seeks to explore the question: On what basis does the medical profession itself seem to assess the value of new diagnostic technologies? It seems reasonable to assume that the direction of change is toward ever more precise diagnosis. It is clear that the medical profession values improving precision and accuracy. Risk, too, is important, for risks are associated with many diagnostic technologies. The use of X-rays, of radionucleotides, or of such techniques as pneumography (involving the injection of air into the chambers of the brain) all pose risks to the patient. We may assume that a new technology will be preferred to the extent that it is more accurate and less risky than what was available before. But what if the two criteria conflict? Moreover, to what extent is the medical profession swayed by considerations of cost in a situation of limited resources?

As part of the general problem of assessing impact, a second question to be considered is the effect of technological change on the availability of care. In other words: How is technological change equated with the health needs of the whole community? [2]

Mass screening for a variety of diseases is increasingly considered a critical aspect of preventive health. Consideration of the use of technology in screening raises certain interesting questions. On the one hand, such extension in the use of technology seems to ensure that the benefits of innovation are widely distributed. On the other hand, there does seem to be a danger of "diseconomies of scale." That is, it may be—and this question is certainly debated in the medical literature—that the large-scale use of a new procedure may provoke difficulties that do not arise when its use is restricted to a few major specialized centers.

II. CASE STUDIES

A. Radiology and Ultrasound in Obstetrics

Between the mid-1940s and the mid-1950s the likelihood of a foetus' being X-rayed increased substantially, for the techniques were increasingly used in obstetric diagnosis. By 1955 about one in seven women who subsequently produced a live child were being radiographed. In a series of papers dating from 1956, Stewart and her colleagues at the University of Oxford demonstrated epidemiologically that X-rays posed a risk of subsequent cancer to the unborn child. The proportion of all live births previously X-rayed *in utero* began to fall from about that time: 1957–1960 has been termed the period of "greatest radiological caution." At the same time radiological techniques were improving: High-kV techniques with intensifying screens, faster films, and other technical improvements resulted in smaller doses of radiation per exposure.

Technical improvement would thus appear to have reduced the risk of iatrogenic cancer. However, leaving aside the undoubted benefits to those who might have been obstetrically at risk, evaluation of the "social risk" of obstetric radiography is complex. The risk to society (equivalent to the economist's notion of "social cost") is considered the product of individual risk (which was reduced by technical improvement) and utilization, or extent of usage. In a 1968 paper, Stewart et al. attempted to assess the interplay of these forces. Taking cohorts of births in the years between 1946 and 1962, and armed with knowledge of prior radiographic exposure, they examined cancer mortality before the age of 10 (1968). How had the risk of cancer mortality associated with obstetric radiography changed relative to the "normal" cancer risk between 1946 and 1962? It appears that although radiography became much safer in the late 1940s, subsequently the proportion of cancer deaths attributable to X-rays fluctuated, no regular decline was recorded, and the rate was roughly equal to those recorded for other causes in under 10 year olds. The conclusion was equivocal: . . . Data . . . neither support the idea of a small but constant increase in the risk of dying from cancer before the age of 10 years after irradiation *in utero*, nor do they confirm a steady trend towards safer obstetric radiography. . . .

The risks and the need for caution having been demonstrated, what has happened since? A recently-published study of eight hospitals typical of the range of hospital practice in 1974 showed that on average 22.7 percent of pregnant women were being X-rayed: Proportions ranged between 8.6 percent in one hospital and 34.8 percent in another (Carmichael and Berry, 1976). The authors commented: "It seems that where a patient attends a hospital with readily available X-ray facilities, these facilities will be used." The effects of the demonstration of risk appear to have had little impact. In one hospital the proportion of pregnant women X-rayed, after rising from 30 percent in 1953 to 39.7 percent in 1955 and then falling to only 11.0 percent in 1961, had risen again to 23.0 percent by 1974. Moreover, according to the authors, this second expansion in usage had not been accompanied by further technical improvement. Since 1961, when Donald and Brown described its principle and use in obstetrics, X-ray techniques to some extent have been in competition with ultrasound examination.

Diagnostic ultrasound is based on the principle that the velocity of transmissions of high-frequency sound waves (beyond the range of human hearing) in a substance depends on its composition. The composition of a substance can thus be studied by examining the transmission of ultrasound through it or alternatively of the echoes produced. These principles were first applied in the 1930s and 1940s in the development of underwater communication (sonar used by submarines in World War II) and methods of detecting flaws in materials. The idea that similar techniques could be used to detect and locate tumors in soft human tissue gave rise to considerable research in the postwar years (Bronzino, 1977). By the early 1950s some success attended these efforts. The many subsequent refinements and improvements have been largely attributed to the increasing sophistication of electronic technology. Ultrasonic techniques have yielded a number of applications in obstetrics, including the diagnosis of early pregnancy, the localization of the placenta, the determination of the number of foetuses, and the monitoring of foetal development. By mid-1972 some 80 commercial sonographs were being used for obstetric purposes in the United Kingdom.

Initial fears that ultrasound would involve some risk of chromosome damage appear unfounded, and the prevalent view is that the technique is entirely harmless (Boyd et al., 1971).

How does the technique rate on accuracy and ease of use compared to alternative methods? These questions seem to be the most discussed in the obstetric and radiological literature. In placental localization, Reed (1973) argues that "the accuracy of the technique is equal to that of most other methods and superior to most." In estimating foetal maturity, Fletcher found that whenever patients had been tested both by ultrasound and radiography, the predictions were in close agreement (1978). In both cases, the ultrasonic technique was compared with others involving radiation risk. In estimating foetal development, an alternative involves measuring the concentration of oestriol in the mother's urine, a technique that is also without risk. In 1967 it was shown that ultrasonic measurement of the foetal head size (ultrasonic cephalometry) gave a quantitative and reliable indication of foetal development and served as a predictor of birth weight. The then-new application was defended thus:

> Oestriol measurements are complicated and the results have not in the past been immediately available to the clinician, in contrast to the result of ultrasonic cephalometry which is a simple technique with the minimum inconvenience to the patient.
>
> Some obstetricians might say that they could give just as accurate a prediction of dysmaturity in two thirds of cases by abdominal palpation alone. They might have great difficulty, however, in detecting an alteration in the growth rate of the baby, and they would not be able to apply an accurate objective standard. (Willocks et al., 1967)

As with many diagnostic technologies, doubt now seems only to surround the simplicity and the accuracy of the technique when applied not by senior radiologists in major centers but by the wide range of staff who may be involved in its mass use in ordinary hospitals. Reed attempted to meet this objection by examining the records of the use of ultrasonic placentography in the 18 months after installation of the equipment in an ordinary district hospital (1973). He concluded that the error (i.e., diagnosis proved wrong by operative findings or by the outcome of labor being at total variance with the ultrasonic report) in a series of 400 tests was only 3.5 percent. This incidence was attributed to errors committed during the course of acquiring experience. Nevertheless, others argue that for ultrasonic scanning to be deployed optimally, there is a need for much greater skill in operation and for an increase in personnel (the technicians) actually trained to operate the equipment (Meire, 1977). Bronzino quoted the American Society of Ultrasound Technical Specialists as estimating that its present 1,000 members will need to be increased to 20,000 to 80,000 within the next decade (1977, p. 143).

Despite considerations of risk and accuracy, radiography and ultrasonic scanning are now used in parallel. Thus at one large hospital (in which over 4,500 women were delivered in the year 1976–1977), 431 women were radiographed, and another 1,900 were examined by ultrasound (on average, 2.7 times each). A study of this hospital suggests that ultrasound could replace radiography to a considerable extent (perhaps half). The reasons for its failure to be so used seem to be the rejection of requests for radiographs made by junior staff not familiar with ultrasound as well as money. Complete ultrasound coverage necessitates a second ultrasonograph (which costs about £10,000 and another £10,000 per annum in running costs). These funds were not available (Fletcher, 1978).

B. Clinical Examination and Mammography in Screening for Breast Cancer

It is now widely accepted that a program of screening can greatly reduce mortality from cancer of the breast in women. There exists a number of diagnostic techniques, of which the most common are simple clinical examination and breast X-ray (mammography). A third technique available is thermography. This technique makes use of the findings that infrared emission depends on temperature and that tumors are hotter. The principle involves plotting infrared emissions from the body under controlled conditions. Although thermography is absolutely harmless, the interpretation of thermograms is difficult, and a great deal of skill is required. Radiologists consider that thermography should never be used alone but always in confirmation of the findings of other techniques.

Let us therefore consider the merits of clinical examination and mammography initially on the basis of accuracy and risk. It should be noted that the usual procedure after screening by whichever method is to refer suspects to hospitals for further tests. If these tests prove positive, a woman will be admitted to a hospital on an inpatient basis for biopsy. The accuracy of a technique is judged in two ways. In the first place, doctors look for a low rate of false negatives, that is, cancers undetected.

But they also look for a low rate of false positives because unnecessary referral can give rise to anxiety, inconvenience, and the possibility of morbidity associated with surgery and anaesthesia. In terms of false negatives, a recent attempt at comparing the accuracy of the two techniques found that mammography was more accurate. The percentages of false negatives in screening a sample of 1,215 women aged over 40 were: mammography alone 26; clinical examination alone 42; combined tests 11. In terms of the referral rate for what proved to be nonmalignant conditions, the results were 5 percent, 15 percent, and 18 percent (Chamberlain et al., 1975). This study, which concluded that neither technique was wholly accurate and that clinical examination was subject to observer variation, was based on a view that the value of mammography had to be proved. In view of its risk (see below) and because of the costs entailed by equipment and specialized staff, the technique had to be proved superior to clinical examination in order to be adopted. Another authority, a radiologist, denied the value of such comparisons (Young, 1975). He argued that a comparison of methods is meaningless because so much depends on the skill of the diagnostician and the amount of care taken and that all available techniques must be used together. Considering thermography, he wrote: "Many workers have shown conclusively that the highest preoperative diagnostic accuracy in breast disease, and the discovery of early malignancy, can be achieved only by the correlative use of all three primary methods." What about the risk posed by exposure to radiation?

> The risk of one or two sets of mammograms with dosage to each breast of between 2 and 6 rads for diagnostic purposes would seem no more than in many other accepted radiological procedures. But in survey work where yearly mammography is done, the question of dangerous levels of irradiation certainly arises. A practical risk threshold of 2 rads per breast has been suggested and it is possible that survey work should be confined to women over 40 which would limit the lifetime of yearly examinations to approximately 30 (1975).

In other words, although mammography is more accurate, it would be risky to do regular checkups by this method other than on women over 40 (who are more but not uniquely at risk).

Most writers seem to recognize that if there is to be a program of mass screening, then cost considerations are relevant. For Chamberlain et al. this conclusion was a major reason to improve the accuracy of mammography. Even Young, who has argued for the use of all techniques, has pointed out that although the diagnostic clarity of mammograms can be improved by "cleaning up," through the use of radiographic intensifiers, these devices are very expensive. At the other end of the scale of technological commitment, two general practitioners, who carried out a trial screening in their practice of women over 25 who accepted an invitation to attend a local clinic, argued the cost advantages of clinical examination:

> The equipment needed for these special techniques is very expensive, however, and staff have to be specially trained. It is unlikely therefore that either mammography or infrared thermography will be available in large enough numbers to screen a large population, at least in the near future. It was these considerations that prompted us to undertake this study using only the simplest equipment, the human hand. . . . (Barnes et al., 1968)

It seems clear that improvements in diagnostic accuracy impose costs: both financial and in terms of risk to the population. But it also seems clear that different representatives of the medical profession make their "trade-offs" in quite different ways. Some seem to argue that a new technology that is both more expensive and more risky has to prove its greater accuracy. Others seem to argue that the objective is the greatest *possible* accuracy and that the fewest necessary concessions should be made. Not addressed, although highly relevant to an effective screening program, is the question of attendance. How much less likely are women to attend hospital X-ray departments than visit their individual general practitioners?

C. Amniocentesis and Screening for Foetal Abnormalities

Current tendencies toward greater emphasis on screening as an aspect of preventive health stem from the desire to reduce both individual suffering and the social costs of many diseases and conditions. Cost-benefit analysis is one aspect of the debate over the effectiveness of screening. Use of the most up-to-date techniques may be considered one means of making the benefits of new diagnostic technologies as widely available as possible, and insofar as there is a "technological imperative" in medicine, it is likely to be manifest also in screening practices. The two previous case studies throw some light on this aspect of the question. It is interesting also that Bronzino, admittedly a bioengineer, looks forward to the day when complete CAT scans will form part of multiphasic screening tests (1977, p. 153).

Nevertheless, it is recognized that population screening involves indirect costs. Certain costs are not related to specific technologies, such as anxiety and disruption arising from a "false positive" diagnosis. Technology-related costs include the possibility of iatrogenically-induced cancer of the breast from repeated mammographies. Moreover, it should be recognized that a technique necessitating hospitalization (or even hospital attendance) may generate a lower rate of usage than one that (although perhaps less accurate) can be carried out by a family doctor. The "effectiveness" of a technique has to be distinguished from its clinical accuracy.

The debate surrounding amniocentesis raises these questions[3] in acute form, and it is referred to here even though, strictly speaking, amniocentesis is not a new "technology." By sampling the amniotic fluid surrounding a foetus, it has been possible, using cytological techniques, to test for chromosomal abnormalities, such as Down's syndrome, since the mid-1960s. The techniques are not easy, and the procedure has largely been restricted to women considered "at risk" (the most common indication being a first pregnancy in a woman over 40).

In late 1972, however, it was shown that foetal neural-tube malformations (for example, spina bifida) are associated with a greatly increased concentration of alpha feto protein (AFP) in the amniotic fluid. At about 16–17 weeks after conception, almost all cases of anencephaly and spina bifida show raised AFP levels. Thus as a *Lancet* editorial commented in mid-1974, "Amniocentesis followed by AFP determination could, in principle, provide a prenatal diagnosis for 90% of all serious spina bifida (and virtually all anencephaly) in ample time for selective abortion." (1, 1974, p. 907)

Amniocentesis is not, as the *Lancet* editorial maintained, "a procedure to be undertaken lightly." It should be preceded by an ultrasound scan to locate the placenta, to ensure single birth, and to estimate foetal maturity. If there is no adequate localization, there is a danger that the needle will cause bleeding, foetal damage, or spontaneous abortion (1 percent risk). If the procedure is attempted too early, it is likely to fail and the risk of foetal damage is increased. However, ultrasonic scanners are not universally available, and the scans require considerable skill in interpretation. Even with the scan (according to *Lancet*), a risk remains.

It was therefore judged that AFP determination should continue to be restricted to women at high risk of bearing foetuses with neural-tube malformations or genetic disorders. Unfortunately, knowledge of the etiology of these disorders is slight, and imposing such a restriction would have reduced the birth prevalence by only about 10 percent.

Wider screening was debated. Laurence wrote, "In view of the seriousness of both spina bifida cyctica and Down's syndrome, with their attendant family problems and the high costs of treatment and care, it might be argued that it would be well worth extending the scope of screening to include a much greater proportion of the pregnancies." (1974)

Indeed, a stronger case (of a kind) could be made for monitoring all pregnancies in Northern Ireland, Wales, and Scotland, where the incidence of such birth defects is about twice the average of England. "However," this author maintains, "such a policy would not be justifiable nor logistically practicable," partly because obstetrics departments and cytological laboratories would not be able to cope with the extra work. Another aspect relates to what can be called "diseconomies of scale": "Inevitably many amniocenteses would be carried out by relatively inexperienced staff, probably without a previous ultrasound scan, with the resultant risk of all sorts of mishaps and almost certainly a greatly increased number of miscarriages."

At the time that Laurence's article was written, clinical research, which subsequently transformed the debate, was in the course of being published. A number of papers published in *Lancet* between autumn 1973 and spring 1974 suggested that neural-tube defects of the foetus are associated with raised AFP levels not only in amniotic fluid but also in maternal blood serum. The concentrations in question are 500 times lower than in amniotic fluid and require extremely sensitive methods of assay. Moreover, for some while, the relationships between the concentration distributions of normal and abnormal were unclear (i.e., at what level should abnormality be assumed). This test, which uses blood samples taken as a matter of course, is without direct risk and seems to offer (in principle) a method of preliminary screening. In 1975 Leighton et al. published tables of AFP-level distributions and settled on a 95 percentile cutoff point: "Findings reported have shown that only a proportion (around 2 percent) of cases with a normal foetus will be above the 95th percentile on repeat estimations."

The recommended procedure involves following two "positives" on this test by an ultrasound scan and then amniocentesis. Consideration of termination (abortion) would follow "positive" amniocentesis. Risks still remain. There remains the 1 percent risk of spontaneous abortion with amniocentesis, and there is the psychological cost to the 2 percent of patients with normal foetuses who will be unnecessarily referred for this test on the basis of blood-level assays. Nevertheless, there is little doubt that the findings published in 1973–1974 (whatever the direct interests of the researchers) greatly reduce the risks associated with screening for neural-tube defects. (As already indicated, powerful interests are demanding the introduction of such tests throughout the United Kingdom.)

Clinical or epidemiological research that specifies the population to be subjected to a potentially damaging diagnostic procedure is an important aspect of reducing the risk of the technique.

III. CONCLUSIONS

This paper has sought to illuminate some of the questions implicit in studying the impact of technological change on diagnostic medicine. What criteria enter into the evaluation of new technologies by the medical profession, and, in particular, how is "risk" balanced against "accuracy"? Is there evidence that medical technology is (or could become) "self-generating," that is, develop according to an internal dynamic having little to do with broader priorities in medical care? Do there appear to be "diseconomies of scale" (problems in the use of technologies/techniques that obtain only with large-scale use), and has the medical profession developed such a notion? What effect will increasing technological sophistication have on the availability of health care, and how cognizant of these effects does the medical profession seem to be?

Leaving aside the impact of economic and political forces, it appears that the rate and the direction of technological change in medical diagnostics are governed by complex internal tensions. It is widely acknowledged that "technological" and "social" conceptions of medicine coexist (McKeown, 1977). It appears that these conceptions are reflected in different attitudes to new and competing technologies within the medical profession. For example, technical criteria of performance (diagnostic precision) imply the correlative use of at least three techniques in diagnosing breast cancer. Some argue that a complete diagnosis must be done. Others seem to suggest that in view of cost, availability, and risk (of X-rays), simple clinical examination by a family doctor is good enough or better. Those who advocate "technological progress" do not ignore the risks associated with many technologies. There is no doubt that "risk" and "accuracy" are always taken into account, although individuals may weigh them differently in making comparisons. But the tension between technological and social perspectives may be manifest also in somewhat different conceptions of "risk" and "accuracy" in the assessment of technologies. For example, at equivalent levels of risk, a conception of "accuracy" (the number of false positives and false negatives in a population examined) may be in conflict with a conception of "social effectiveness" (which would take account also of different proportions of the population at large who subject themselves to examination) for comparing techniques.

Through the interplay of these various perspectives, diagnostic technology does change. As elsewhere, it seems to change both through the modification of technologies and the introduction of different ones. But there is no *continuing* improvement in either accuracy or safety (despite the enormity of investment in biomedical R&D), as the obstetric radiology example shows. Moreover, reduced risk to the individual (through technical improvement) may be negated at the social level by expanding (less discriminating, less skilled) the use of a technique to which some risk still attaches. The amniocentesis example shows that advance through the reduction of risk may follow less from technical improvement than from (research that leads to) the precise specification of the target population on which the technique will be used. Even when a technology, in terms both of accuracy and safety, seems to be better than an older technology, replacement can be relatively slow. This lag may be reflected in comparing ultrasonic with radiographic techniques in obstetrics, on the basis of which it was suggested that (in the United Kingdom at least) lack of resources, on the one hand, and professional lack of awareness, on the other, may explain the extent to which obstetric radiography has persisted.

On the basis of the evidence presented, it seems difficult to perceive any process of "self-generation" or "internal dynamic" in this area of medical technology. And yet we cannot be sure. The CAT scanner (which many regard as almost entirely irrelevant to medicine, as distinct from medical research) may epitomize a new form of technological dynamic in this area. Indeed, it is interesting that the availability of the scanner seems to be putting the ultrasound technologists on the defensive. A recent article on ultrasound in the *British Journal of Radiology* (Meire, 1977) contained a prediction that CAT would not *eliminate* the need for ultrasound on the grounds of cost, safety (CAT uses X-rays), and accuracy: "Early results from our department suggest that the potential diagnostic accuracy for both techniques is not greatly different for most abdominal organs." The defensive posture in the face of this glamorous new machine can be illustrated by the argument that refers to the enormous sums invested in R&D on computed tomography: "If similar sums were poured into ultrasound research and development, the position might be rather different."

What about the effects of technological change on the availability of health care? Leaving aside the drain on the limited resources of a state medical system that very costly instrumentation (and the requirement of employing associated technical/maintenance staff) may represent, an aspect of this problem relates to the possibility that technological "progress" (implying both safer and more accurate diagnostic techniques) may increase *inequalities* in the receipt of medical care. In the first place (as Russell's work showed for the United States), new technologies are likely to be available first in major centers (or perhaps in more affluent regions). In the second place, they are likely to be used skillfully in those centers. In general, increasing sophistication implies increasing centralization. In other words, geographical inequalities may be accentuated. Social inequalities, too, may be exacerbated partly because the middle class generally makes better use of health services (Carter and Peel, 1977). But it may also be that innovation specifically conduces to the interests of effective and rational consumers. For example, congenital malformations of the central nervous system correlate with a pronounced class gradient in the United Kingdom (Registrar General, 1978). AFP screening involving amniocentesis and termination (if the mother wishes) could eliminate many of these births. In Scotland, 27 percent of married women in Social Class I did not present themselves for care until after the 20th week of pregnancy. This figure rose to over 40 percent of married women in Social Class V[4] (1973 data: Brotherston, 1977). In other words, we may anticipate a further concentration of congenital malformations in Social Class V as a result of presentations too late for amniocentesis and safe termination. It is indeed proper to ask "Cui Bono."

NOTES

1. The distinction between *technological* and *technical* change is commonly made in studying the economics of innovation. The first term means the "advance of technology" (that is, the generation of new methods or products); the second means "an alteration in the character of the equipment, products and organization which are actually being used" (Mansfield, 1968).
2. I do not deal with the relationship between the prevalence of diseases and the inventive effort related to their diagnoses and cure.
3. It also raises ethical questions that are not considered here.
4. In British official statistics, social class is defined on the basis of groupings of occupations: I (professional workers, major employers), II (minor professional workers, managers), III NM (nonmanual-skilled and white-collar workers), IV (semiskilled workers), V (unskilled workers). Married women are classified on the basis of the occupations of their husbands.

REFERENCES

Banta, D. "Public Policy and Medical Technology: Critical Issues Reconsidered." Chapter 5.

Bice, T. W. "Regulation of Capital Investments of Hospitals in the United States: Certificate-of-Need Controls." Chapter 4.

Barnes, S., et al. "Mass Screening for Cancer of the Breast." *Lancet* 1 (1968), 1417.

Boyd, E., et al. "Chromosome Breakage and Ultrasound." *British Medical Journal* 2 (1971), 501.

Bronzino, J. D. *Technology for Patient Care.* St. Louis: C. V. Mosby Co., 1977.

Brotherston, J. "Inequality: Is It Inevitable?" In C. Carter and J. Peel, eds., *Equalities and Inequalities in Health.* London: Academic Press, 1977.

Carmichael, J. H. E. and Berry, R. J. "Diagnostic X-rays in Late Pregnancy and in the Reonate." *Lancet* 1 (1976), 351.

Carter, C., and Peel, J., eds. *Equalities and Inequalities in Health.* London: Academic Press, 1977.

Chamberlain, J., et al. "Validity of Clinical Examination and Mammography as Screening Tests for Breast Cancer." *Lancet* 2, (1975), 1026.

Department of Health and Social Security. *Report of the Supply Board Working Group.* London, May 1978.

Fletcher, E. W. L. "Is Foetal Radiography Really Necessary?" *Lancet* 1 (1978), 600.

Freeman, C. "Economics of Research and Development." In I. Spiegel-Rösing and D. Price, eds. *Science Technology and Society.* London: Sage, 1977.

Fuchs, V. "The Growing Demand for Medical Care." *New England Journal of Medicine* 279 (1968), 190.

Griliches, Z. "Research Costs and Social Returns: Hybrid Corn and Related Innovations." *Journal of Political Economy* (Oct. 1958), 419.

Iglehart, J. K. "The Cost and Regulation of Medical Technology: Future Policy Directions." *Milbank Memorial Fund Quarterly* 55, 1 (1977), 25.

Kervasdoué, J. de. "Are Health Policies Adapted to the Practice of Medical Care?" Chapter 2.

Laurence, K. M. "Screening for Disease: Foetal Malformations and Abnormalities." *Lancet* 2 (1974), 939.

Leighton, P. C., et al. "Levels of Alpha-Fetoprotein in Maternal Blood as a Screening Test for Fetal Neural Tube Defects." *Lancet* 2 (1975), 1012.

McKeown, T. *The Role of Medicine: Dream, Mirage, or Nemesis.* London: Nuffield Prov. Hospital Trust, 1968.

Mansfield, E. *Economics of Technological Change.* New York, 1968.

Meire, H. B. "Radiology Now: Ultrasound-Current Status and Prospects." *British Journal of Radiology* 50 (1977), 379.

Office of Technology Assessment (U.S. Congress). *Development of Medical Technology: Opportunities for Assessment* (August 1976).

Reed, M. F. "Ultrasonic Placentography." *British Journal of Radiology* 46 (1973), 255.

Registrar General. *Occupational Mortality 1970–1972.* London: OPCS, HMSO, 1978.

Russell, Louise B. "The Diffusion of New Hospital Technologies in the United States." *International Journal of Health Services* 6, 4 (1976), 557.

Schmookler, J. *Invention and Economic Growth.* Cambridge, Mass: Harvard University Press, 1966.

Stewart, A. and Kneale, G. W. "Changes in the Cancer Risk Associated with Obstetric Radiology." *Lancet* 1, (1968), 104.

Willocks, et al. "Intrauterine Growth Assessed by Ultrasonic Foetal Cephalometry." *J. Obs. Gyn. Brit. Comm.* 74, 5 (1967), 639.

Young, G. B. "Mammography and Paraclinical Examination of the Breast." In T. Lodge and R. E. Steiner, eds. *Recent Advances in Radiology*. Edinburgh: Churchill, 1975.

Chapter 8

A Systems Approach to Delivery of Care in Health and Disease: Its Impact on Clients

John C. M. Hattinga-Verschure

1. OBJECTIVES AND METHODS

The question of how to improve health in a population is not identical with the question of how to improve the health-care system. The second approach is wider and may include a study of the various kinds of care that are practiced by individuals for the improvement, maintenance, or restoration of their health. Under the names of self-care, self-help groups, cover care, or mutual aid, and so on, these kinds of care-delivery systems outside the realm of the official professional health-care system have become popular in the last few years, especially in the United States. A vast reservoir of powerful influences on health and disease seems to be available in the population. If developments in this field are favorable, influence on the existing professional health-care system may be profound. Thus in a conference on innovative aspects of the health services, a study of these phenomena cannot be omitted.

This chapter does not describe the status of self-care or self-help groups because the subject has been covered in numerous publications that have appeared in this field in recent years. Because less attention has been paid to the theoretical background of care delivery, this contribution is devoted to that subject. It reports the work of the author in this field since the early seventies (1, 2).

The method used consisted mainly of conducting inquiries of long duration into various kinds and ways of health-care delivery by individuals for themselves, by members of groups, and through numerous relationships that characterize the professional health-care delivery system in the Netherlands.

It should be emphasized that the results presented are not the reifications of imagination or conceptualization but represent concrete findings derived from analyses of what actually happens in the numerous situations in which care is delivered. Because the various kinds of care delivery proved to be more or less interrelated, a systems approach was adopted to cover this extensive field.

The work was restricted to the basic levels of *actual* direct delivery of health care. The overhead structures of organization and policymaking have not been included in the analyses. However, it should be recognized that those activities have sound foundations in the realm of possibilities, values, habits, and behavior.

Based on the systems approach chosen, four objectives have been delineated:

1. to *clarify* the multitude of phenomena in a complex cluster;
2. to *create order* by constructing models by means of which the many subsystems and peripheral systems can be analyzed;
3. to *explore* underdeveloped areas in terms of knowledge and policy;
4. to develop a more equilibrated and *comprehensive plan* of health-care delivery with the help of a systems approach.

Governmental policies concerning the health-care system have been restricted entirely to the professional care delivery subsystem. Practically no attention has been paid to the other fields of care delivery that emanate from the population.

2. THREE SUBSYSTEMS OF CARE DELIVERY

In health care there are three subsystems, which, for the purposes of this inquiry, have been designated self-care, cover care, and professional care. These kinds of care delivery are essentially different. The factual observations and argumentations that have led to the decision to divide care delivery into these subsystems were developed by the author in his publication on caring phenomena (2) and have been omitted here for the sake of brevity.

2.1. Self-care

This kind of care delivery covers the self-fulfillment of individual needs. A characteristic of self-care is the shortest possible chain between the provider of care and the recipient, for both are one and the same person. Much of a person's self-care is connected with survival and health in an indirect way. Care needs and the means of satisfying them relate in the first instance to the various physiological processes connected with sustaining life itself: hunger/eating; stress/rest; cold/warmth; danger/defense. Many aspects of physiological self-care are comparable to animal behavior. Most probably, human self-care behavior is rooted in instincts developed during evolution in the animal world. It is largely of genetic origin. Thus it is called natural or unnatural, depending on the survival value of an individual's behavioral pattern. Know-how is not of the cognitive type. It is largely inborn and may well be the result of evolutionary selection over the course of millions of years. Environment may have a strong impact on self-care behavior. Through culture and social structures, values and habits have taken shape that influence the self-care behavior of individuals in certain times and places. These kinds of self-care, designated *basic self-care,* are omnipresent.

In our society much interest seems to be directed toward another level of self-care: the conscious, programmatic attention to conditions of health and what measures individuals can take with the help of modern health sciences and technology. These activities have been designated *programmatic self-care* because they constitute the subject matter of mass-market publications (hundreds of books in this field have been written in the United States) and educational programs. In addition, tools for "lay" people have been produced in order to help individuals determine whether they have normal blood pressure, no sugar in their urine, and so on. Programmatic self-care tends to take over some health-care activities that were performed by health professionals, mainly, general practitioners. The development of the natural and social sciences has yielded information on self-care that can be used to increase the competence of basic self-care so that this pursuit can be lifted from prescientific approaches to a scientific method, as was the case with medical care about a century ago.

2.2. Cover Care

Cover care is comprised of care delivery that individuals, belonging to a (small) group, give to one another. The most basic example of a cover-care group is the family in which parents and children, together with other relations, have mutual care relationships. The defining characteristics are:

Care is given by members of a group on the basis of reciprocity;
the main motivation of care delivery lies *outside* the provider; it is the well-being of "the other";

the chain between the provider and the recipient of care is short and direct; no geographical or organizational distance exists.
the roles of provider and recipient are interchangeable; at one time one is a provider, at another time one is a recipient of care;
the care relationship is comprised of a bundle of interactions, such as parent-child or other family relations, neighbors, friends, companions at work, and so on.
the provider and the recipient of care know each other as persons, not merely as "cases";
cover care is emotionally warm. That is why this name was chosen for this kind of care in 1972 (1).

Examples of cover-care groups are numerous: the family, a group of friends, neighbors, and a group of people who suffer from the same chronic disease or share the objective of restoring their health. Essential to the classification is the notion that individuals are in some sense *companions.* (This statement should not be turned around. Companionship does not mean that people necessarily form cover-care groups.)

From these observations it will be clear that self-care and cover care are manifestly different. To call them both self-care, in contrast to professional care, would blur a justifiable distinction. The words *self-help* and *cover care* may give rise to confusion. Cover care seems to be based on forces of loyalty and other fundamental aspects of human interrelationships. Sociobiology may provide insight into their roots and fundamental aspects by studying the group behavior of various species of animals. The benefit accruing to an individual who provides cover care is of a dialectical nature. In helping "the other," one derives emotional satisfaction, feedback about one's personality, and so on.

Cover care may be divided into two subgroups: heterogeneous and homogeneous cover-care groups.

In a heterogeneous group the participants have different care needs and demands. Examples are neighbor groups, composed of sick or disabled people and strong people who may perform a variety of tasks, and the family, whose needs and demands may vary according to their status as parents, children, or grandparents. Heterogeneous cover-care groups are apt to reflect greater age differences among members and tend to have more extensive patterns of other relations than do homogeneous cover-care groups.

Homogeneous cover-care groups are based on the same care needs and demands of members. The fact that they experience the same kinds of needs creates a feeling of solidarity and provides a trustworthy network for the exchange of advice and help. Examples are a club of good, old friends, in some cases—working parties in small enterprises, a religious group. In recent years great influence and healing capability have been attributed to specific cover-care groups, for example, breast-amputation groups, alcoholics and other addicts, and groups of obese people. Gardener and Riessman (4) have provided an impressive list of such "self-help" groups and agencies in the United States.

Attention has been exclusively directed toward homogeneous cover-care groups. The medical profession has begun to recognize that there exists an incipient method of health-care delivery that has *not* emanated from professional medical knowledge but operates by know-how and draws on forces derived from various resources of life. However, because a systems analysis has not been applied to all the components of the care-delivery systems, little attention has been paid to the possibilities of new kinds of heterogeneous cover-care groups. Examples include "complementary-function" couples and "complementary-function" groups formed by disabled persons. A disabled individual may be deficient in one or more functions, but other functions may be intact or even strengthened by the compensatory mechanisms of the body. The combination of two disabled people who have lost two *different* functions may exercise all the functions that are present in one healthy individual. The classical picture of such a complementary couple was painted by the famous sixteenth-century Flemish painter Pieter Breughel, whose landscape shows two men walking: a blind man, pushing a cart, accompanied by a lame man. Neither would be able to take the walk without help from the other. Today, most probably, we would provide both of them with nurses. Care would be expensive, and the patients would be dependent. But as a complementary-function couple their situation ameliorates and would improve further as they develop cooperative behavior. This option may be available to larger groups under a multitude of conditions. It may prove to be the best way to care for an ever-increasing percentage of old and disabled people. Much imagination and research are necessary to develop this option.

From these observations it will be clear that for cover care as well as for self-care, a division between basic care and programmatic care will be of use in developing sociopolitical activities in health-care delivery.

2.3. Professional Care

The characteristics of professional care are:

Care is given by people who received special training that enabled them to obtain specific certificates;

a direct relationship exists between the kind and the quantity of care delivered and the payment made for such services by the recipient or an agency that acts in his or her behalf;

the chain linking the provider and the recipient of care is long, in a longitudinal and in an organizational sense;
the roles of provider and recipient are *not* interchangeable. Both parties may develop typical role behavior that results in a cleft in their relationship;
the care relationship is the essential one. Other relations that may develop between the provider and the receiver materialize by chance or are extraneous;
the provider and the recipient of care need not know each other as persons;
professional care tends to be emotionally cool because it is characterized by a businesslike approach. It may easily become cold and commercialized.

The descriptions of the various subsystems of caring refer to *typical* situations. Although atypical circumstances, such as emotionally warm professional care or cold cover care, may exist, they can only be clarified by studying the motives, the attitudes, and the behavior of such providers. Apart from atypical circumstances, mixtures of the subsystems also occur. However, for reasons of brevity, no further attention will be paid to them in this paper.

The subsystem of professional health care may be divided in various ways, for example, preventive professional care, curative professional care, and so on. In Western society criticism of professional health-care systems is increasing. Although medical technology continues to develop, the results—in terms of the health of the population as reflected in the statistics of various countries, including the Netherlands—do not represent improvements. *Medical nemesis,* the term coined by Ivan Illich, reflects the reaction to this finding. It has become evident that much criticism is rooted in the secular *shift* in *epidemiology.* Whereas the technological approach has been successful in diagnosing acute diseases, two other categories of unhealthiness have increased in Western society: psychosocial disturbances of health and multipathological disturbances affecting elderly, chronically ill, or disabled people. These groups have grown tremendously because of the success achieved in combatting the causes of death to which people used to be subject in earlier stages of the life cycle.

The growth of these groups suggests that new approaches of cure and care are required. To adhere to the technological system effective in treating acute diseases could prove not only unsuccessful but harmful should overmedication constitute a mode of treatment.

Criticism in the Netherlands is slowly increasing, as many signals suggest. Disgruntled patients have begun to form local groups. On a national level, several agencies have been established, for instance, patienten-beraad and clientenbond. Among young intellectuals in the big cities, criticism is widespread.

Even among medical students, seldom conspicuous for their revolutionary attitudes, action to bring about change in medical education has been taken. Critics have used approaches that are common to advocates of change in similar situations: protests, publications that present extreme solutions and alternatives that may result in throwing away the child with the bath water, overstress the "human" approach to patients, and underestimate the healing powers of modern medicine, and so forth. Often the proposed innovations have been described in terms of a shift from the "medical model" to the "social model."

If the objectives of innovation are formulated in terms of health status (and not in terms of efficiency or financial responsibility), it may become apparent that curing is no longer the only objective: Innovation of care is the central concern.

3. RELATIONSHIPS AMONG THE THREE SUBSYSTEMS OF CARE DELIVERY

Self-care is the only subsystem that exists on its own; notably, animals that lead solitary lives are entirely independent.

We may learn from sociobiologists how much interaction that has the appearance of mutual care exists among animals living in groups. Most impressive is the care that nest birds give to their young. Many aspects of cover care are present. Concerning the cover care that can be discerned by observing the singing birds in our gardens, we have the strong impression that care is "emotionally warm" and that the parents give care "with great love" and "devotion"—attributes of human cover care that we may be projecting to the animals.

A phenomenon of care delivery is that the more an individual is able to support himself or herself, less cover care is delivered. From nature, unspoiled by the complications that may arise from human consciousness, we learn that the basic kind of care delivery is self-care. When the self-care is deficient, it can be completed by cover care.

With the help of some simple models, the various relationships among care-delivery subsystems can be visualized. The sizes of the circles are rough approximations of the magnitude of care delivery (Figure 8.1).

For many animals (and humans) living in solitude, the only kind of care is self-care. For animals, self-care is always sufficient; otherwise they could not survive. (See Figure 8.2.) For humans living in solitude, self-

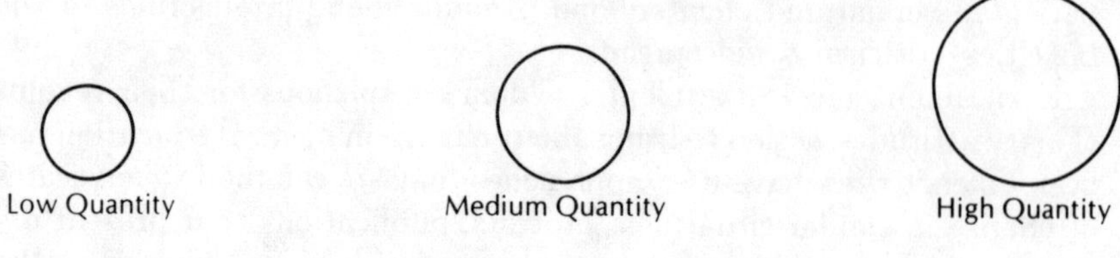

Figure 8.1.

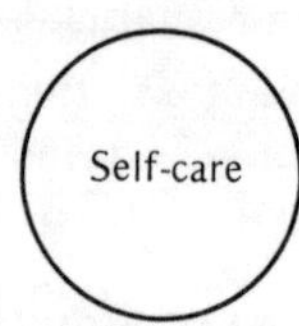

Figure 8.2. Care model for animals and humans in solitude.

care is not merely a matter of "instinct" but also of habit and choice. Thus self-care may be sufficient (as in the case of animals), but it may also be deficient or underdeveloped (Figure 8.3).

The situation of care delivery for a young child: Self-care is underdeveloped. Complementary cover care is large and diminishes as the self-care of the child develops. (See Figure 8.4.)

Both self-care and cover care develop normally and in equilibrium with one another.

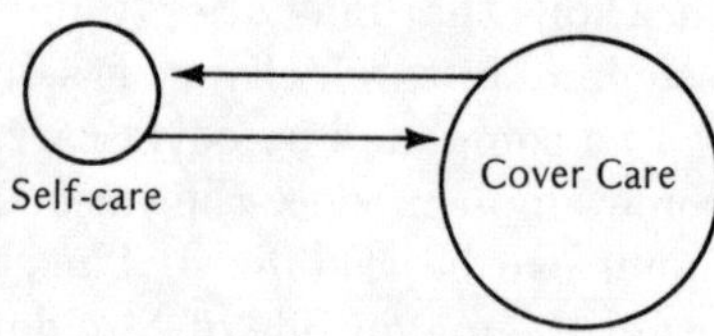

Figure 8.3.

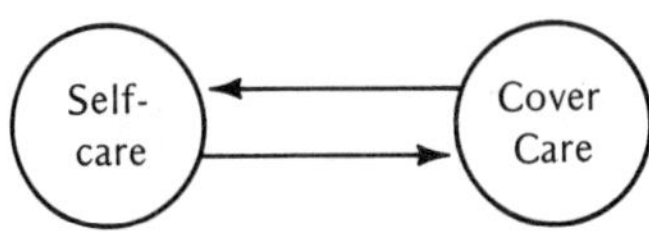

Figure 8.4. The care pattern in a normal family.

Only when one feels *incompetent* to care for some disturbance of one's health and when others believe that their cover care may be deficient, one decides to seek help from the professional subsystem. A general practitioner pays a visit to the home of a patient and gives advice to the family and the patient. Now the three systems are in operation and interacting with one another. The model is illustrated in Figure 8.5. The various relations are different. Some are care relationships, others are financial, and so on.

If the patient is taken to a hospital, the picture, as illustrated in Figure 8.6, changes considerably. Self-care and cover care are largely superseded by care dispensed by the nursing staff. In the northern countries of Europe, cover care in hospitals is virtually ruled out. Most care delivery is taken over by members of the professional subsystem. This approach may be necessary for a short period of acute illnesses. However, if in the course of caring, an individual suffering from a chronic illness or a handicap is not encouraged to restore his or her natural care-delivery activities, a most vital mechanism of human life could be damaged. The sense of life itself could be affected.

In Western society old age is usually considered a handicap. With increasing age, cover-care relations tend to diminish: The great mobility of

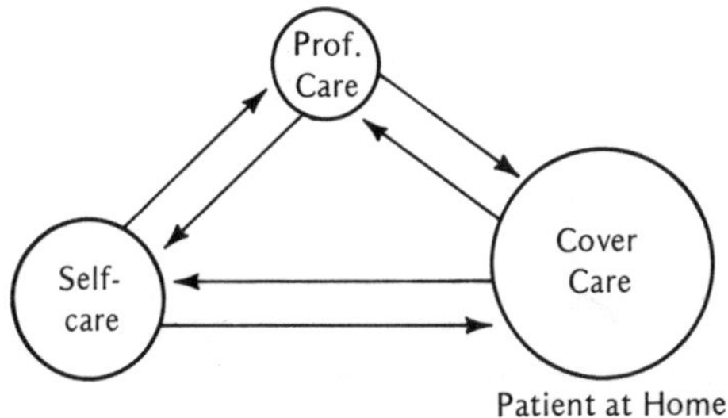

Figure 8.5.

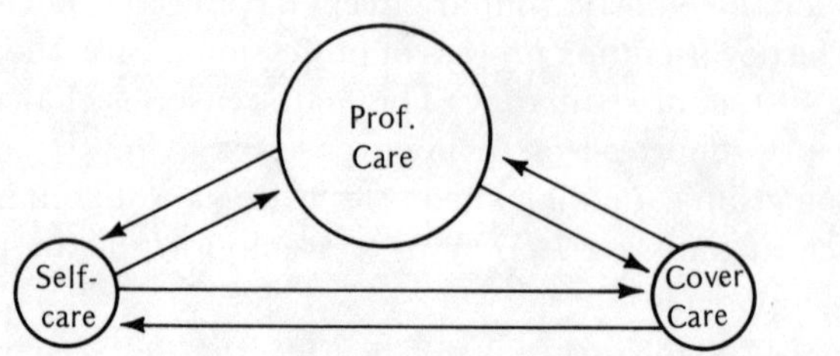

Figure 8.6.

the population contributes to the dissolution of the family; friends and relatives die; one becomes more or less an alien in one's living quarters (Figure 8.7).

It would be most sensible to try to reverse cover-care atrophy. However, Western society has devised a different solution. If the stability of life is endangered in old people, they are usually put into institutes for the elderly (Figure 8.8).

We know about the untoward effects of institutionalization called hospitalization syndrome. From many observations made in nursing homes

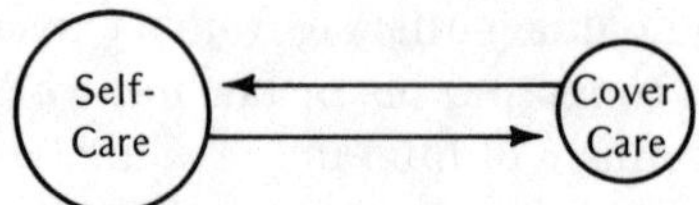

Figure 8.7. The care model for old people: cover-care atrophy.

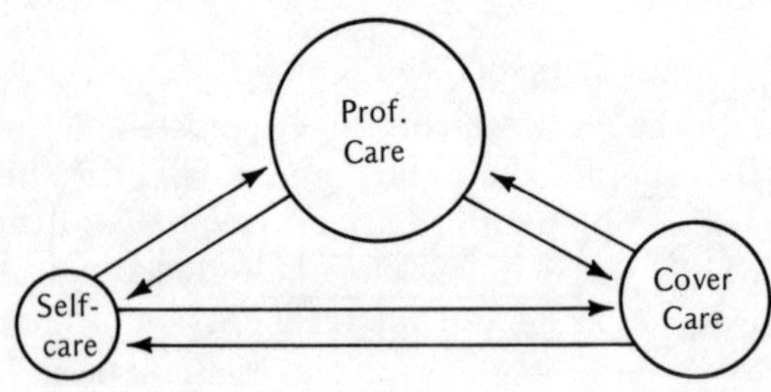

Figure 8.8.

and homes for the elderly, similar effects have been reported. When enmeshed in the never-ending process of professional care, the clients of our health-care system are unhappy. The main reason is that they feel useless and empty—deprived of their purpose for living. It is evident that caring for something and for someone as well as for oneself is essential for sustaining spirit and satisfaction, or so a majority of the population in the Netherlands reports.

Not only overmedicalization but overprofessionalization and overinstitutionalization in general seem to be the major defects of the system of health care. In the Netherlands, the elaborate social-security system is largely responsible for this development. Overinstitutionalization is now recognized by the government as an undesirable development. Measures to combat this situation have been taken but will be effective only after the passage of many years. The overprofessionalization of health care has had a serious psychological impact. People have become convinced that only a diploma means competence: No diploma, no competence. Self-care and cover care are considered prescientific approaches to the delivery of health care, the mastery of which involves no diploma. Thus they have been depreciated in the public consciousness as "amateurism."

When highly-complicated medical technology is emphasized, the "lay" person begins to feel incompetent about handling the maintenance of his or her health. Individuals then tend to rely for health care on the professional subsystem.

4. INNOVATION IN CARING FOR HEALTH

The nucleus of all innovation in health care seems to be the restoration of cover care and self-care.

4.1. Objectives of Health Care

One might ask if this conclusion means that planners and policymakers should manipulate the public in this direction. Although the choice of a health-care system should be a public prerogative, the choice should be based on the most complete information available and the clarification of alternatives. Thus the main tasks to be pursued consist of more research about care and caring and the transmission of more information to the public.

First, the objectives of health care should be reconsidered. For example, a discussion is going on in the Netherlands about whether the crite-

Table 8.1 Satisfaction with Health Situations ($N = 4{,}637$)

Health Situations, as Stated by Individuals	*Extremely Contented* (%)	*Very Contented* (%)	*Contented* (%)	*Rather Contented* (%)	*Discontented* (%)
Healthy	35	37	23	4	1
Occasional acute illness	21	40	28	9	2
Chronic or recurrent illness	11	22	30	19	18
% of total	21	31	27	12	9

ria of the medical profession or the needs of clients should prevail. Table 8.1 suggests the lack of correlation between these objectives. (5)

In a random sample of the population in the Netherlands, the interviewees were asked to classify themselves according to their health conditions. In a subsequent question, they were asked to rank their levels of satisfaction with their conditions of health. The answers are given in percentages in Table 8.1. It is surprising that many people who reported rather poor health declared themselves extremely or very contented with their situations. (52%).

5. SELF-CARE IN THE NETHERLANDS

In general, self-care among the population of the Netherlands is considered low. The reasons have already been discussed. Although the government is emphasizing the development of health education, the promotion of self-care seems to be more a matter of *motivation* than of information (6, 7, 8).

The "state of the art" has recently been described by Rouwenhorst (3). The Netherlands Heart Foundation is active in promoting habits that should conduce to the prevention of heart disease. Interest in self-care is slowly increasing in the professions. For example, the society of community nurses, in evaluating the objectives of their profession, produced a report (9) recommending the promotion of self-care and cover care. Although the medical profession in general is either oblivious or reluctant to encourage innovative forces in care delivery, Kuiper is promoting such change in social medicine (10).

Testing self-care capacity is restricted to ADL (Activities, Daily Life). The results are used to determine whether handicapped or elderly people should be hospitalized. Standardization of decisions is lacking; each institution tends to use its own set of criteria. Self-care opportunities in institutions (hospitals, nursing homes, homes for mentally-retarded people, and others) are few. In general, the client is subject to professional care.

Criticism of health care that engenders infantile dependences among clients is stronger among professionals than among the clients themselves. The term *therapeutic environment* suggests the development of a strong trend that could culminate in giving clients more responsibility for their treatment and more respect for their wants and wishes. This environment may be favorable for the development of self-care (and cover care) of hospitalized people. Research concerning the correlation between more self-care (and cover care) of institutionalized persons and their happiness is in the pilot phase only. (11) Preliminary results suggest that the life force of an individual may be reinforced if he or she is actively involved in caring for himself, herself, and others instead of merely being cared for.

6. COVER CARE IN THE NETHERLANDS

Huygen has studied the importance of stable families for the health of children in a Dutch community (12), a study that is especially interesting in light of the increasing number of divorces. During the seventies, the divorce rate doubled in five years, calculated per million inhabitants. On the other hand, in more and more areas, especially in large cities, local committees have begun to care for their own inhabitants and living quarters. Often initiated to devise plans for housing, rehabilitation, and so on, they have developed, in a number of cases, provisions for cover care. The development of homogeneous cover-care groups in the Netherlands lags behind developments in the United States, which can be ascertained from the recent inventory compiled by Gardner and Riessman.

The development of cover care among elderly people and among patients in nursing homes is being investigated by students from the institute with which the author is affiliated. They have found that cover care provided by family members for their relative in nursing homes is usually discontinued within three months of the patient's admission (13).

7. SUMMARY AND CONCLUSION

Innovation in health care should not be restricted to the *structure* of the professional subsystem. To do so would diminish and perhaps silence innovative signals that are being emitted from the health subsystems of self-care and cover care.

A brief review of the circumstances that conduce to these innovations in the Netherlands has been given, and a theory of care delivery, based on long-term inquiry by the author, has been presented. Hypotheses have been confronted with empirical data, and the situations under investigation have been discussed.

The final conclusion of the author is that innovation in health care should be pursued in *two* ways. One way is to innovate *structures* within the professional care-delivery subsystem. Until recently, this approach absorbed the attention of planners and governments. However, a second approach now seems to be indispensable: the innovation of habits, skills, and values concerning self-care and cover care for the health of the population–in short, establishing a new *health culture* in the Western world. The author hopes that this innovative approach to health care will not be confused with policies that can be described as "tapping community resources" or "mobilizing voluntary work."

REFERENCES

1. Hattinga-Verschure, J. C. M. "Ontwikkeling van zorgcriteria voor herstructurering van de gezondheidszorg." *Het ziekenhuis* 2 (1972) 500.
2. ———. *Het verschijnsel zorg.* Lochem, Neth.: De Tijdstroom, 1977.
3. Rouwenhorst, W. *Leren gezond te zijn?* Alphen a/d Rijn: Samson, 1977.
4. Gardner, A., and Riessman, F. *Self-help in the Human Services.* San Francisco: Jossey-Bass, 1977.
5. De leefsituatie van de Nederlandse bevolking 1974. Deel 1: *kerncijfers.* Table 19.8. 's-Gravenhage: Staatsuitgeverij, 1975.
6. Haes, W. F. M., de, Schuurman, J. H., and Sturmans, F. "Gezondheidsvoorlichting-en opvoeding. "Gedragsdeterminaten." *Medisch Contact* 31 (1976) 385.
7. Schuurman, J. H., Haes, W. F. M., de, and Sturmans, F. "Verandering van gedrag." *Medisch Contact* 31 (1976) 421.
8. ———. "Opvoeding tot gezond gedrag." *Medisch Contact* 31 (1976) 475.
9. Alleen samen. *Discussienota over de toekomst van het Kruiswerk.* Utrecht, 1977.
10. Kuiper, J. P. "Het zal onze zorg zijn." Assen/Amsterdam: Van Gorcum, 1976.
11. Reijners, B., et al. *wie zorgt daarvoor? Een oriënterend onderzoek naar*

aanknopingspunten voor welzijnsverbetering in verpleeghuis Vreugdehof Amsterdam. Report. Utrecht: Institute of Hospital Sciences, 1978.

12. Huygen, F. J. A. In: *Waar gaat onze gezondheidszorg naar toe*. Bilthoven: Ambo, 1977.
13. Beernink, W. A. M. Gespreksgroepen met familieleden van verpleeghuisbewoners. Nederlands Tijdschrift voor Gerontologie (1977), no. 8.

PART III

Institution Building and Administration: Issues in Centralization/ Decentralization, Innovation, and Responsiveness

The chapters that constitute Part III of this volume have two common themes: how to go from seeking and developing change to managing it and how to overcome the numerous behavioral, attitudinal, and organizational obstacles to change? The speed with which medical technology is diffused has hardly any parallel in the history of health policy as far as social and organizational engineering are concerned because of the numerous cultural and political traditions of those involved in or affected by social and organizational changes.

Furthermore, unlike developmental strategies for launching medical technology, those for implementing change or for restructuring service delivery are in short supply irrespective of whether innovations are mandated by the central government or initiated by health advocates in the periphery. The problems and the difficulties of achieving interorganizational and intergroup cooperation and collaboration—essential prerequisites for social and organizational innovations—abound.

Both cooperation and collaboration connote a broad spectrum of positive relationships that has engendered widespread popularity as well as ambiguous meanings. With respect to restructuring the delivery of services, do we mean "architectural coordination" when providers and clients are spatially close to one another, when they get together on a regular basis, or when service providers form an association to promote their interests? Do we mean "substantive coordination" when patient-clients receive services in some kind of sequence and order that is designed to treat their medical problems? Can we have the latter without the former? Do we get "substantive coordination" only through "architectural coordination"?

With respect to cooperation and collaboration in center-periphery relationships maintained for the purpose of implementing national policy, do we achieve cooperation more easily through reforms that follow a bottom-up or a top-down strategy? Can cooperation and collaboration be coerced, mandated, or elicited by the use of economic and financial sanctions? Do certain cultural traditions sustain collaborative as well as voluntary efforts, and are these traditions the major prerequisites for innovation? How do we overcome established reward structures, civil-service rules, and financial incentives or disincentives that so often work against cooperation in policy implementation and inhibit the integration of human services? These and other questions are examined in the following cases.

In his comparative study of labor-initiated innovations in the Federal Republic of Germany, Italy, Sweden, and the United States, Frieder Naschold points to the similarities of problems encountered in the field of work-caused diseases and the different responses that they have evoked in different social and political environments. The existence of two competing paradigms for the setting of standards in the field of occupational health and safety largely impeded progress in the past. Recent responses to resolving the dilemma of competing conceptions reveal major differences between the approaches pursued by European countries and that followed by the United States. Four essential aspects of those approaches are identified and evaluated critically.

Naschold's analysis leads him to pose the following questions: What are some major policy innovations in the field of occupational health and safety (OHS) standards that contrast with the traditional strategies of state intervention? What are the goals, instruments, vehicles of interorganizational cooperation, and features of "worker medicine"? In particular, how do labor-union innovations and worker-oriented health conceptions compare with traditional conceptions of industrial medicine? What are some of the conditions that conduce to the introduction of innovating strategies for OHS at the plant level? Who are the agents? What are the barriers and the opportunities, and what instruments are being used? These and other questions are of central concern to Frieder Naschold.

W. Robert Curtis and Duncan Neuhauser report on the experiences of managing change when no additional external funding was available for the delivery of mental-health services in a community in the state of Massachusetts. As a result of developing theoretical insights into the nature of mental health, a strategy of deinstitutionalization was pursued. The authors critically examine the widely differing kinds of problems encountered and the equally wide-ranging responses of political and professional forces resistant to or supportive of these changes in both the community and in the state. Organizational/structural innovations in service delivery capable of (a) responding to the need for providing geographical services and (b) fulfilling appropriate organizational functions require flexible organizational mechanisms in order to succeed. Evaluative criteria for assessing flexibility are discussed extensively.

In their report on Swedish efforts to achieve coordination, Ragnar Berfenstram and Ragnhild Placht examine the theory and the practice of coordinating national policy on health and social services at every governmental level and stage of service delivery. They also analyze the implementation of health and social services in the field. The Tierp Project serves as a laboratory for assessing different kinds of prerequisites for successful coordination. It included the implementation of several specific programs in the social and health area and involved a network of governmental officials and an array of service providers that differed in professional roles, status, and prestige, as well as authority. The authors critically examine the different kinds of problems that arose, which either were of an organizational or an interpersonal nature.

The paper by the late R. G. S. Brown critically examines the difficulties and the problems encountered in introducing a comprehensive planning system for the English health and personal social services in 1976. Particular attention is paid to the priorities set for the National Health Service, to the workings of new structures for health-services management and decision-making processes, and, finally, to norms for resource allocation.

By drawing attention to the significance of organizational development in ensuring innovations, A. S. Härö evaluates, from the perspective of a national planner, progress made in Finland toward implementing innovations that were mandated by law. The strengthening and the expansion of primary care through adequate and equitable distribution were the chief goals of Finnish policy. To carry out corrective actions, a change in central-local government relationships was also required. After relating the basic constraints of the Finnish political and health-care systems, he discusses the balance that was struck between the need for the centralization of decision making over goals and control instruments and the need for decentralization in a country that has sustained strong traditions of local autonomy. Knowing what health policy the country had pursued in the past and its experiences with strict national norms and standards seems to be the best predictor of the direction of new legislation.

From the perspective of local implementors of the national public health-insurance program in the Federal Republic of Germany, Christa Altenstetter examines the impact of national and state decisions on health-insurance funds in several communities by drawing on recent field work. She is interested in the normative and the empirical aspects of Selbstverwaltung in German health-insurance funds. What are the effects of national and state legislation on Selbstverwaltung? Who are the main decision makers in a general sickness fund, and what are their responsibilities? What do local insurance funds do? Can they be innovative and responsive to local needs and circumstances? These are some of the questions that she explores in her contribution to this volume.

Chapter 9

Two Roads Toward Innovation in Occupational Safety and Health in Western Countries

Frieder Naschold

In the decade 1965–1975, intensive efforts to improve the existing systems of occupational safety and health (OSH) were made in numerous Western industrial nations. In most cases, three factors can be considered the driving forces behind these developments:

urgent political demands made by the labor movement;
the growth of health and safety hazards;
noncosting reform strategies proposed by government parties and state agencies.

In most countries the predominant innovative response consisted of extending the previous system of administrative standards and controls undertaken by professionals within the enterprise. Parallel to and partly against this main trend, the labor movement in some of these countries succeeded in carrying through quite different basic innovations in the area of occupational safety and health that included increasing control over production processes and the mobilization of employees in behalf of new forms of OSH.

The main emphasis of this chapter will be on the juxtaposition of these two kinds of innovations, with special consideration given to labor-

I thank Dr. Hugh Mosley and Dr. Peter Tergeist for their valuable assistance.

initiated innovations in the Federal Republic of Germany, the United States, Italy, and Sweden. But first the underlying problems of policy resulting from work-caused diseases as well as the fundamental paradigms of OSH will be discussed.

1. THE DEVELOPMENT AND THE EXTENT OF WORK-CAUSED DISEASES

The development and the extent of work-caused diseases can be demonstrated by using the example of political debate and scientific research in the United States. The implementation of the standard relating to the Occupational Safety and Health Act—"that no employee shall suffer material impairment of health or functional capacity"—requires sufficient information on the extent, development, etiology, and pathogenesis of work-caused diseases, for this novel approach expands the existing system of workmen's compensation with respect to occupational safety. This extension is the result of a successful political debate conducted by an offensive labor movement, the expanded definition of OSH, and subsequent administrative reactions. The accompanying problems and conflicts can provide rich illustrative material for the incipient development of an OSH system in Germany after the passage of the Work Security Act.[1]

A. Work-related diseases caused by physical, chemical, biological, and stress-related impairments that have developed or been recognized only in the last decades are more complex and complicated than traditional work injuries and require novel and preventive strategies. Their etiologies are characterized by the intense or prolonged exposure to health hazards and to isolated and specific noxious substances that are often not only confined to places of work. Their pathogenesis is often protractive, cumulative, and irreversible; their progression affects sensory perception, respiration, specific organs, and the central nervous system. For these reasons they deviate from the traditional problems associated with occupational safety and health hazards.

B. For the same reasons the ways of reporting OSH only detect the "tip of the iceberg" of these developments. Recent field studies have revealed a high incidence of these diseases—in one sample of 900 persons, almost 40 percent, whereas only 2 percent were reported to the Occupational Safety and Health Administration (OSHA) by the enterprises concerned, and only 30 percent were reported to accident insurance companies. In part, the reasons for these striking discrepancies inhere in problems of diagnosis. The explanation can be traced to the simplistic health and safety standards of the OSH system, defects in the entrepreneurial-reporting system required by OSHA, and avoidance strategies adopted by individual companies.

C. The reasons for this unexpected increase in work-caused diseases relate to dynamic economic developments, that is, the massive growth of chemical health hazards and noxious physical elements (noise, heat, radioactivity) and the psychosocial stress factors associated with methods of continuous production and the intensification of work. According to recent studies, about 80 to 90 percent of all carcinomas are caused by environmental factors, and 50 percent of these can be attributed to work-related hazardous substances. This finding corresponds to the parallel development of industrialization and to increases in the cancer rate. The other most acute diseases—heart disease and chronic bronchitis and emphysema—are, to a large extent, traceable to the causes noted above. If these findings are extrapolated, we can expect, within the next two decades, a rapid increase of these diseases, discernible genetic effects, and decreasing life expectancy.

D. Quite "naturally" the burden resulting from these developments falls most heavily on the lower social strata: Industrial workers are suffering from work-caused impairments at a rate ten times higher than that recorded for professionals in the tertiary sector. Despite the protection afforded by OSH, about 90 percent of the direct, indirect, and hidden costs of these impairments are borne by the employees themselves, whereas the "business-controlled compensation safety establishment," using a multitude of defense and avoidance strategies, pays only about 10 percent of these costs.

The gulf between the threat, the extent, and the progression of these work-caused hazards, on the one hand, and the existing occupational safety and health-delivery system in the United States, on the other, has increased to such an extent that it can no longer be bridged by gradual changes in existing safety standards and control procedures but requires an effective and far-reaching system of *preventive* medicine. The implementation of such a system depends less on the increasing stress generated in the work place than on the outcome of conflicting social forces.

2. TWO PARADIGMS COVERING THE SCIENTIFIC SETTING OF STANDARDS IN OCCUPATIONAL SAFETY AND HEALTH

Concerning strategies to change the existing OSH delivery systems, which will be discussed briefly with reference to the United States, of central importance is the development and the establishment of protective occupational safety and health standards and effective procedures for their implementation.[2] According to the OSH act, standards are developed by an independent scientific research team whose findings are implemented through administrative, juridical, and political measures. The scientific core of these standards can be characterized as follows:

the material problems of OSH are defined as value-neutral, professional (technical and medical) problems independent of their societal settings;
they are examined by neutral and independent experts assigned on the basis of the division of labor;
the experts' evaluations reflect scientific standards of decision making;
the aim of scientific evaluations is the formulation of objective standards that approximate the truth.

This process of setting standards is characterized by two components: first, an implicit or an explicit elaboration of paradigms that illuminate the causes and the process of overcoming work-caused impairments, and, second, the specification of concrete standards based on these paradigms.

Since the turn of the century, when the first political debates about the subject occurred, the problems of occupational safety and health have been approached by the use of two competing paradigms. For Paradigm I, accidents are caused by various psychological and physiological characteristics of "accident proneness" in the individual and by behavioral "unsafe acts." Work-caused diseases are traced primarily to an "extreme susceptibility" of the sensitive part of the population that has a disproportionate sickness rate. The strategy designed to overcome work-caused impairments, a strategy that results from these basic assumptions, involves transferring, dismissing, or not hiring the "sensitive" in accordance with the judgments of the scientific experts and the maintenance of the existing structure of work.

For Paradigm II, the basic assumptions of Paradigm I constitute a "myth," the behavioral consequences of which are rejected as a strategy of "blaming the victim." Paradigm II perceives accidents as caused mainly by unsafe conditions of the work process and work environment. Accordingly, diseases are traced to objective perils, such as exposure to hazardous substances at the work place and factors of the work environment. It rejects the protective measures of Paradigm I as "misleading" and "impracticable" and proposes to overcome health and safety hazards by a preventive approach that stresses secure technology and effective industrial medicine.

In specifying the assumptions of the latter paradigm, two competing concepts can be distinguished. Concept I (threshold limit values–TLV) proceeds from the assumption that the body's reaction to exposure to hazardous substances is shaped by certain threshold values that allow the distinction between "safe" and "unsafe" levels of exposure to toxic substances. The marginal exposure level can be defined as the guiding standard (TLV). The scientific validity of Concept I is subject to dispute because of the complexity of illnesses that makes it difficult to prove causal connections and the fact that standards are usually agreed upon as a compromise among scientific, legal, administrative, and economic considerations. The protective function of TLV is considered problematic because of the necessarily tedious process of standard setting and especially because norms can control work-caused exposure levels but not the individual health conditions of affected persons. In its strategic consequences, the concept can lead to preventive measures that can be applied in occupational safety and health. On the other hand, major deficiencies are obvious:

Few economic incentives and/or pressures have been generated for the introduction of protection in accordance with the standards of OSHA;
the increasing gap between the rapid spread of toxic substances and the process of standard setting;
personal selection as the predominant mode of protection.

In view of the low preventive impact of occupational safety and health measures devised according to the TLV concept, the alternative Concept II recognizes the necessity of developing "a totally new and revolutionary approach" toward diseases caused by exposure to toxic substances at the work place. This concept proceeds from the assumption that in the case of carcinogens, "the zero threshold is likely enough to be true to warrant decisions as if it were true." [3]

From this assumption three central elements can be deduced:

for carcinogens, zero concentration (no detectable level of exposure) is demanded together with strong administrative controls ("use-permit system");
for other toxic substances, the demand focuses on "premarket testing" in connection with safety limits for similar groups of substances;
the rigorous restructuring of hazardous work places and work processes, the development of "safe substitutes" in connection with the unequivocal rejection of any quid pro quo between safe jobs, on the one hand, and company profits and employment, on the other hand.

Even if the scientific validity of Concept II cannot be established with respect to the assumption of zero concentration, the standards that have been developed—although based on less rigorous scientific requirements—are sufficiently safe and do not countenance great risks. In addition, high protection can be afforded by employing simple and "conservative" criteria, the reversal of the burden of proof, an accelerated process of standard setting, reduced administrative-control expenditures, and a strong emphasis on the internalization of social costs at the plant level. On the other hand, a precondition for its functioning—and this precondition suggests a potential weakness of the concept—is the strong deployment of political power as a substitute for scientific-investigative procedures. Despite this potential weakness, Concept II represents a "new and revolutionary approach" toward far-reaching improvements in occupational safety and health.

3. COMPARATIVE PERSPECTIVES ON STATE INTERVENTION IN OCCUPATIONAL SAFETY AND HEALTH

The political elites and state apparatuses in the aforementioned countries were forced to react to the increasing demand for a preventive reorientation toward occupational safety and health. They responded by trying to add some innovative elements to the strategies of intervention that they had been pursuing for some time.

The traditional occupational safety and health-delivery system rests on two pillars: State agencies or, by delegation, intermediate agencies, such as the "Berufsgenossenschaften" or private "Normenausschüsse," try to set standards, establish norms, and proclaim goals. State and semistate institutions supervise work conditions and enforce standards and norms in order to guarantee the protection of workers. This system of standard setting and supervision was a great invention in the nineteenth century, but it did not fulfill its objectives, not even with respect to the traditional health and safety hazards generated by early industrialization. It has proved to be even more deficient under present working conditions.

The occupational safety and health laws enacted in the 1970s generally contain three major provisions that could constitute major policy innovations:

A. Broadening the goals of occupational safety and health by extending the definition of occupational diseases to include work-caused diseases and by shifting the focus to preventive instead of curative action;

B. establishing instruments (occupational physicians and safety officers) on a large scale through the introduction of professionals at the plant level in order to fulfill these new goals;
C. building interorganizational cooperation among professionals, company officials, and the local works councils—representatives of trade-union locals and state and semistate agencies.

When compared with the United States model, some essential differences can be noted. These differences characterize European, especially West German and Swedish, strategies toward occupational safety and health protection.

1. A qualitatively and quantitatively more elaborate administrative steering structure, coupled with a relatively stronger trade-union position both at the plant level and in collective bargaining, that can provide the social power basis for occupational protection.
2. The first difference produces a more flexible strategy designed to implement protection by using administrative control agencies that can advise and admonish by employing their powers of discretion instead of using the relatively inflexible strategy of supervising by means of imposing rigid standards, administrative sanctions, and legalized coercion.
3. A system of implementation that is close to or even situated at the plant level, based on the assumptions of "voluntary compliance" and "self-regulation," as opposed to a system of external controls in which protective standards are set externally.
4. A strategy of overcoming work-caused impairment that is strongly oriented toward industrial medicine and ergonomics, in contrast with a primarily engineering orientation toward occupational safety and health. From a summary evaluation of how close the occupational safety and health delivery systems both in European countries and in the United States have come to their goals after having expanded the traditional strategy of state intervention to include the aforementioned innovative elements for about eight years, the following overall assessment can be made:[4]
   i. The administrative steering structure and the social power base are not sufficiently strong to ensure the implementation of occupational safety and health standards to any significant degree.
   ii. Curative reaction still predominates over strategies of overcoming work-caused impairment through the internalization of costs, the restructuring of work, and technological innovation.
   iii. The fact that companies only formally fulfill or even totally ig-

nore administrative OSH standards prevented significant overall improvement. Instead, an increase in work-caused impairments suffered by a large part of the working population has been recorded.

iv. The pressing problems of occupational safety and health in small enterprises, in sectors with weak union representation, and in unorganized plants are ignored in public debate and proposals directed toward political mobilization; these enterprises and plants play a prominent role especially in the United States social system.

v. The resulting disillusionment experienced by the political groups supporting reform led them to demand even more far-reaching reforms: Preventive work safety and health policy requires at least greatly expanded research oriented toward critical problem areas and guided by the criterion of a prevention-oriented policy (in the United States NIOSH is the agency responsible for such a research strategy); more emphasis on health standards as well as on the general-duty clause and the development of this approach as an alternative to the prevailing emphasis on work safety with engineering-oriented approaches to the problem; workmen's compensation coverage for work-caused illnesses; increased and adequate training of physicians and safety experts in occupational health, together with a work place-oriented, preventive team approach on the part of various experts; obligatory plant-level medical services for the primary prevention of occupational illness, not only treatment, or secondary prevention, or, in the case of small businesses, joint health centers; a switch in priorities from local counseling to legal enforcement backed by sanctions.

Although evaluations of new state occupational safety and health programs in Europe suggest a less pessimistic prognosis than that suggested by the American case, one can judge the German, Italian, and Swedish programs failures if the fulfillment of their original aims is used as the criterion of evaluation.

4. LABOR-UNION INNOVATIONS IN THE OCCUPATIONAL SAFETY AND HEALTH SYSTEM IN COMPARATIVE PERSPECTIVE

The attempts of the labor-union movements in these countries to make occupational safety and health issues part of the collective-bargaining process and to mobilize workers at the factory level for a policy of collective self-help represent significant sociopolitical innovations. Such strategies have taken different forms and developed in varying degrees in individual countries. On the whole, they correspond to the assumptions of Paradigm II and Concept II and strive toward a general political mobilization over the issue of occupational safety and health and toward the active participation of workers with the aid of professionals and state agencies. The most far-reaching concepts and practices are to be found in the Italian labor-union movement. Similar interesting developments in occupational safety and health can be observed in the United States, Sweden, and the Federal Republic of Germany.

The development of worker medicine (in contrast to industrial medicine) since the late 1960s was the result of massive criticism by northern Italian workers of work organization and its impact on health and skill levels.[5] Metal workers in particular criticized the "value-neutral objectivity" of scientific work organization and industrial medicine that support the interests of the employers in a one-sided way. Thus the evaluation and the classification system for defining jobs, work norms, and pay was criticized as well as the traditional conception of industrial medicine. They became the object of industrial conflict at the plant level and the critique of these traditional approaches led to the development of an alternative worker-oriented health conception, that is, worker medicine.

Initially, progressive physicians, psychologists, technicians, and other scientists attempted to propagate their findings through the medium of established union-education programs. They called on workers not to trade their health for money but to struggle against health hazards in the work place. Nevertheless, the relationship between scientists and workers remained the same. The scientists had their own language, which was difficult for others to understand. They assumed that the workers were unable to recognize industrial health hazards and that they needed the better informed intellectuals to enlighten them about their true interests.

Only in the second phase did the typical characteristics of worker medicine begin to crystallize. It began with a union-sponsored survey of problems in the plant. Questionnaires that were prestructured by the scientists but enabled the workers to formulate independent answers about health problems in the plant were administered to the workers. The result was a "Report on Health in the Factory" (1973), which formed the basis for further union health-policy proposals.

The essential characteristics of worker medicine include the following:

a. The observation of the plant work situation and its harmful effects on workers is recognized as an effective investigative method. In this way the subjective factor of individual well-being in the plant can be transformed into a concrete concept of stress and can provide the basis for the articulation of workers' demands.

b. The determination of harmful work situations takes place through the medium of collective discussions and evaluations. The standards of industrial medicine can be modified, and potentially harmful situations can be ascertained. Generally, however, the traditional measurement of a harmful situation by the practitioners of industrial medicine and the collective evaluation of stress by the workers are considered equally valid and supplement one another.
c. Collective evaluation is undertaken by a homogeneous group of workers, the smallest unit in the enterprise, who share the same work environment and therefore are exposed to comparable health hazards.
d. Worker medicine derives its basic premise from the deficiencies of plant health care: "There is only one group in the factory that has a direct interest in protecting the health of the workers—the workers themselves." Hence the corresponding principle of not delegating responsibility for health protection to individuals who merely administer the health interests of the workers.
e. These features of worker medicine require a language that can be used within the plant as well as a new system designed to disseminate information on the health situation in the plant. The former was attempted by producing handbooks in which the work situation in the plant was analyzed on the basis of the workers' experiences with its impact on their health. The second required permanent control of the work environment by means of a work-environment register (in which various stress factors and their effects are described), a medical-statistical register (in which health problems at the group level are recorded), and an individual health-hazards book.
f. Because those aspects of work organization and work environment that cause illness have become the object of union policy, worker medicine focuses directly on the elimination of the causes of sickness. Of course, a precondition of such a policy is a change in labor-union wage policy, which has been oriented toward financial compensation for dangers confronted and stress experienced on the job.

Worker medicine has now become the common platform of all important labor unions in Italy. First realized in the large plants of the metal and chemical industry in northern Italy, it has been implemented in large plants in other industries through collective-bargaining agreements.

Bologna offers an example of how this approach can be integrated into a regional health system. In 1971 the Bologna Health Office, working with the labor unions, founded a preventive medicine group, which, at the request of the workers in a company, provides assistance in analyzing harmful health conditions in the plant. The prevention group and the union jointly convene a plant meeting at which workers and health experts discuss symptoms of disease and causal conditions that may exist in the plant. Thereafter they formulate a set of health-security demands to be presented to management and devise a strategy to gain their acceptance. This regional joint effort has led to a heightened consciousness about health that conduces to primary prevention.

For a long time, problems of occupational safety and health were only of secondary importance for the American union movement.[6] Wage issues and job protection were of primary importance for this union movement that is characterized by declining membership, organizational fragmentation, and lack of perspective. In light of the high value placed on occupational safety and health by rank-and-file workers, union leaders and top management have joined forces to propound the notion that mobilization to resolve such problems could lead to a power shift in the system of industrial relations that would be disadvantageous to both sides. There is also the traditional ambivalent attitude of American unions toward the state. This ambivalent if not indifferent attitude is reflected in the general approach of the large unions in the AFL-CIO: central management of the legally-established structures for intervention, administrative processing of problems, and a minimal commitment of personnel and other resources to the problem of occupational safety and health. This behavior syndrome may well account for the limited impact of the Occupational Safety and Health Act.

In contrast to the widespread bureaucratic lethargy of the large labor unions, a few smaller, more progressive unions that have succeeded in expanding their memberships in industries that have experienced a high degree of risk were able to achieve some spectacular successes in the course of militant confrontation. Militant locals raised qualitatively new demands for the improvement of work conditions and were able to achieve many of their demands in alliance with public-interest groups (e.g., the Health Research Group in New York and regional COSH groups).

The occupational safety and health policy of the Oil, Chemical, and Atomic Workers Union (OCAW), under the direction of their health and safety expert, Toni Maccochi, has received international recognition. Evidence attesting to the observation that the harmful effects of certain work processes and materials cause new forms of work-related diseases, such as sterility and specific genetic defects, that relate to increasing automation, rising profits, increases in carcinomas and in noise levels, and declining employment. Corresponding relationships can be uncovered between psychological stress and the intensification of work in continuous and integrated forms of production.

Recognition of these relationships can be discerned in radical demands for occupational safety and health. The unmistakable impact on work-related safety and health problems of the growth and modernization strategies pursued by individual industries may make the problem of hazardous work environments and materials a dominant issue and could become the motivating force that strengthens the American union movement. The basis for such a policy of occupational safety and health must be built on the experiences accumulated by the militant rank and file in alliance with progressive professional groups who may espouse differing political orientations. Thus in addition to a series of internationally-recognized model contracts based on OSHA, a number of outstanding rank-and-file activities, training programs, internship programs, and joint research institutes are of international interest. Local 688 of the Teamsters developed a multitude of activities directed toward "self-education" and the "self-organization" of work. Based on a limited budget, a seven-point action program was drawn up, a situation analysis was written, and a list of demands was presented to management—a procedure that has become a practice. The rubber workers union negotiated a contract that provides for a research program to be financed by the company and jointly developed in a school of public health. The results of the program are to be made available to the appropriate OSH committee. These results will then form the basis for further occupational safety and health recommendations. Also of importance are numerous training activities that the UAW and the OCAW regularly conduct. These activities are open to all members of the unions. The OCAW has also proposed an internship program designed to provide physicians trained in industrial medicine with experience of the industrial world. Through this program physicians paid by the union and the company become familiar with unions and with workers' problems during the course of their formal medical training. In this way "management doctors" are to be balanced by doctors sympathetic to the problems of union workers.

In Sweden, in an entirely different political and economic setting, personnel and institutional innovations have been devised in order to realize, through the participation of the affected workers, the far-reaching occupational safety and health goals set by law.[7] A central role is played by the educational safety supervisor, who is selected by the local union organization. The education programs are conducted jointly by the union, the employers' organization, and the state Work Safety Office. The unions are making considerable efforts to strengthen the influence of the safety supervisor. In their judgment, it is important that the safety supervisor acquire practical experience that should enable him or her to initiate and implement appropriate measures in each situation, economic knowledge in order to be able to counter the economic arguments advanced by management during negotiations, and technical competence that should extend to taking measurements in the work place. As a work safety expert of the LO explained, the acquisition of technical competence makes it possible to attain work-safety expertise. It is not yet clear to what extent these training goals have been fulfilled nor whether advanced training has exerted the intended impact on practices in the work place.

In contrast to the Federal Republic of Germany, employees or their representatives play central roles in the entire occupational safety and health system. Because of the relatively large number of safety supervisors, the employees have the potential to function as members of a report and warning system. The perception of work problems as safety and health hazards requires no delegation of responsibility by the employees; observation can take place inside the system itself. The sensitivity of the system to stress is thereby heightened.

The direct participation of the employees facilitates the integration of occupational safety and health measures in the remedial systems that exist in almost all work contexts. Furthermore, because the elected safety supervisors are often part of such work contexts and hence are familiar with the remedial systems, it is easier to coordinate necessary protective measures within such systems. When the employees become active participants in the occupational safety and health system and not merely its objects, protective measures can be devised, refined, and institutionalized without friction.

The central role of the employees in the occupational safety and health system involves formal decision-making competence in all questions of occupational health and safety in the work milieu. The predominant role of the employees and the relatively generous allocation of financial resources for the improvement of the work milieu can lead to decisions that conduce to the mutual interest of employees and management. Possibilities seem to have materialized in Sweden but not in the Federal Republic. These developments have led to a relatively more responsive occupational safety and health system in Sweden. As experience shows, measures designed to effect the enlightened interests of both parties have failed in the Federal Republic because of the power relationships that prevail in plants.

In the Federal Republic, employee-oriented, rank-and-file-focused strategies directed toward medical protection are comparatively underdeveloped. There is a small number of such initiatives.[8] On the one hand, the position of the unions as they struggle to preserve labor power has become more tenuous because of the economic situation and social insecurity; on the other hand, because the pace of work has intensified to an unprecedented extent, medical protection remains a significant political problem. But procedures designed to separate issues pertaining to health hazards from those relating to wages are being devised. Further progress is evident in the increasing recognition that is being accorded to occupational safety and health issues by the employees and their elected representatives:

1. Within the works councils, occupational safety and health interests, which have traditionally been regarded as only of marginal importance, are receiving increasing attention. This attention is manifest in the increasing number of workers who are participating in union-training programs and the increasing participation of works-council chairpersons in such training programs.
2. Increasing activities, for example, concluding plant agreements about the concrete tasks to be performed by works physicians, are filling gaps in existing legislation and regulation and ensuring that laws will be observed.
3. In individual, although probably few, plants, works councils have developed their own definitions of hazards in the plant and have intervened with works physicians.
4. The main bottleneck for the medical occupational safety and health system relates to the difficulty of generating information about all those problem areas in which nothing "objective" can be measured. Affected persons frequently hesitate to articulate complaints about work-related impairments because of anxiety that they might lose their jobs. There is no lack of data-processing machinery and machine-readable questionnaires that could facilitate the acquisition of knowledge. But there is a dearth of trusted persons in the work area who are knowledgeable about stress problems and can initiate action. An important development in this direction was the promulgation of a demand articulated at the 12.IG-Metal Union conference in 1977. The union demanded that the safety supervisor in every work area be elected by the workers themselves instead of being chosen by managment—the current practice.
5. Finally, the new generation of industrial physicians should be mentioned. Although still a minority, this group recognizes that the achievement of preventive medicine in the work place is less dependent on their legal status, although that status is essential to the fulfillment of their functions, than it is on their continuous and cooperative relations with employees whose health is at stake.

The limitations evident in state interventionist policies in occupational safety and health and the development of rank-and-file-oriented policies, especially by the labor unions in Italy and Sweden and, although less effective, in the United States and the Federal Republic, suggest the potential for innovation in policies designed to ensure genuine primary prevention, provide remedial measures, and control competence.

NOTES

1. F. Naschold, Arbeitsschutz in den USA und präventive Sozialpolitik; dp-78/17, Internationales Institut für Vergleichende Gesellschaftsforschung, Wissenschaftszentrum Berlin, Oktober 1978; reprinted in WSI-Mitteilungen 1978/10, pp. 16 ff.
2. N. Ashford, *Crisis in the Workplace* (Cambridge, Mass.: MIT-Press 1976); D. Berman, "Death on the Job," *Monthly Review Press,* 1979.
3. *Ibid.*
4. F. Naschold, Arbeitsschutz in den USA and präventive Socialpolitik, *op. cit.,* pp. 4 ff.
5. H. Abholz et al., Die Entwicklung der Arbeitermedizin, also Beitrag zur Humanisierung der Arbeit in: WSI-Mitteilungen, 1978/11; RV/78-9 IIVG-Papers, WZB.
6. F. Naschold, Arbeitsschutz in den USA und präventive Sozialpolitik, *op. cit.,* pp. 22 ff.
7. F. Hauss and F. Naschold, Arbeitsschutz und Sozialpartnerschaft in Schweden; Informationen und Thesen, IIVG-papers, WZB, Oktober 1978.
8. H. Kühn and F. Hauss, Entwicklungstendenzen im medizinischen Arbeitsschutz; Thesen; PV/78-5, IIVG-papers, WZB, Mai 1978; reprinted in Jahrbuch für Kritische Medizin, Argument-Sonderband, Berlin West, 1978.

Chapter 10

Reorganizing Human Services in Massachusetts

W. Robert Curtis and Duncan Neuhauser

In 1955 the high tide of the old era of mental-health care in the United States was reached. Most mentally-ill paitents were hospitalized in large, isolated, state-owned mental institutions. The typical features of this system were 2,000-patient facilities, two-year stays, and per-patient budgets so low that treatment was infrequent. When treatment did occur, it was often based on a theory of mental illness that focused on the failure of personality development assumed to be caused by childhood trauma. In the mid-1950s new drugs were marketed that controlled extreme moods and socially-unacceptable behavior. Theory changed. Mental illness was redefined as either a psychological or a biochemical failure.

More patients could be taken out of the state hospital and returned to their communities, which would provide settings for the resolution of problems. This idea formed the basis for the Federal Community Mental Health Center Act of 1963 that proposed establishing centers for populations of 75,000 to 250,000 throughout the United States. Deinstitutionalization followed and continues to this day.

By 1967 the Massachusetts State Department of Mental Health had divided the state into 7 regions and 40 areas, as shown in Table 10.1. One of these 40 areas is *Taunton.*

Taunton took this one unique step farther by creating *community human-service centers* serving communities of about 10,000 people. It was assumed that the mental health of individuals is affected by their relationships with their friends, family, and neighbors (their *social networks*). Helping people requires working with their social networks, and this kind of work could only be accomplished by providing services within small communities.

Table 10.1 Four Levels of the Department of Mental Health's Organizational Structure

Date	*Level of Organization*	*Population*
Prior to 1900	State of Massachusetts Department of Mental Health Central Office in Boston	6 million
In place in 1968	7 regions	1 million (approximately)
In place in 1967	40 areas	75,000–250,000
In place in 1976 (In Taunton only: 10 community human-service centers)	600 communities	about 10,000

THE ROLE OF THEORY

In 1970 the Taunton area of Massachusetts received its mental-health care from a traditional, large state mental hospital. Acute medical care was provided for this area by independent, entrepreneurial doctors, as exemplified in the American pattern of medical practice. The changes that we will describe have taken place outside the acute care services.

Although only 50 miles from Boston, the officials who presided over this area of the state had not found it easy to attract professional workers or new sources of funding. Instead of waiting for the government to fund its professional staff, Taunton developed an experimental program and established a community and neighborhood structure to provide the resources with which to help people experiencing difficulties in living.

Within this experimental program, new theories were put into practice. Mental illness was treated first as a social problem and then as a psychological or physical problem. One was not separated from the other as a prerequisite to specialized treatment. This approach required that mental-health care be provided by people who were knowledgeable about a patient's social network and environment, knowledge that could not be acquired at an isolated state hospital. Nor could this kind of care be given in a mental-health center serving 100,000 people. It had to be dispensed in local community centers serving 10,000 people or less, where the staff knew or had access to nearly everyone in the community. The approach involved the redefinition of mental health to include all human services. As an initial step in this change of focus, patients became clients and were recognized as partners in rather than objects of the change process.

Another theoretical basis for new practices relates to the definition of problems. People have problems that usually do not fit into neat categories corresponding to current service structures. For example: A 17-year-old has dropped out of school, is unemployed, has no job skills, and is awaiting trial for selling drugs; his parents are separated, and he is depressed. Under the present system, it is difficult or impossible to bring together various professionals to help solve his problems because police, teachers, job counselors, and mental-health therapists are associated with different government bureaucracies.

The community human-service centers developed in Taunton departed from a narrow focus on treating mental health and adopted the broader focus of a human-service event, which includes (1) the individual client and the social environment; and (2) the public organizations providing human services.

Using resources released from the mental hospital, instead of new state appropriations, 10 human-service centers (HSCs) were established at the community level in the Taunton area between 1972 and 1976. Patients were released from the hospital, reducing the census and making possible the transfer of resources.[1] Inpatient beds decreased from 160 to 60. The remaining beds at the Taunton State Hospital served the other 6 areas in Region 7. (See Table 10.2.) State resources for maintaining the centers, particularly funds for personnel, came from the state hospital.

Table 10.2 Taunton Area Census Reduction

	1960	*1970*	*1971*	*1977*
Taunton State Hospital Patients	2,000	1,000	160	60 Taunton unit
			840	800 other units

In 1970 the region's 2,000-bed hospital was divided so that each part could serve an area. The total number of beds was reduced to 1,000, and a mental-health center was planned for each of the 7 geographic areas. Taunton's unique feature was an even more decentralized approach. A human-service center was provided for each community of 10,000.

MANAGING THE CHANGE

Managing the change required theories and practices designed to solve a number of organizational problems. For example, no new money was available. Consequently, Taunton's plan was based on moving state workers out of the hospital along with the patients. This effort was impeded by rigid civil-service rules that required the holder of a position to retire or quit before his or her job classification could be changed to conform to changed responsibilities.

The change provoked the opposition of the labor union. The union preferred to have its members work together in one place. Management was able to convince some union members that the change would confer mutual benefits. A few workers volunteered for the new assignments. They discovered that community work was more exciting than hospital duties and encouraged others to follow their examples. The union did not object to transfers that were initiated by its members. The union feared that deinstitutionalization would mean job losses. However, because the centers generate strong community support, it may turn out in the long run that the establishment of human-service centers is the safest way to protect jobs.

It was soon recognized in Taunton that many providers of human services were not employed by the State Department of Mental Health. A survey reported that 20 percent of the adults living in the Taunton area were willing to volunteer approximately four hours a week to help troubled people in their communities. Based on these responses, "problem-solving teams"[2] of volunteers were formed to provide direct services to those who would otherwise have been hospitalized. On the assumption that community volunteers would be better able to respond to clients' social networks, community involvement was encouraged, and a campaign was launched to raise money from community members who began to perceive the human-service centers as vehicles for their participation—a notion never inspired by the state hospital.

Another resistant force emerged from the arena of politically-active interest groups that usually lose influence when decentralization occurs. These groups consisted of mental-health associations, professional organizations, mental-retardation associations, and private providers. The enthusiasm generated in local communities was sufficient to counter this resistance. In effect, one political constituency was replaced by another, the only difference being that the new constituency is a general rather than a special interest group. In the long run, its interests might not be focused sharply enough to sustain political efficacy and provide a counterbalance to special interest groups.

Increased structural complexity was another problem that resulted from the Taunton plan. A fourth level (community) was added to the state bureaucracy that encompassed three levels (state, region, and area). Many argued that the existing structure was clumsy and inefficient and that the addition of 600 small units throughout the state would compound the situation.[3] A similar argument held that the disadvantages of requiring management to deliver comprehensive services at the community level outweighed the benefits that could conduce to clients and staff from instituting this kind of a system.

It was evident that a new kind of organizational structure was required to respond to these problems. A structure was needed to coordinate general social services based in community human-service centers and to provide access to more specialized services, such as income maintenance and hospitalization, located at other organizational levels within the state. By creating a balance between centralized and decentralized authority, services could be shaped to the general needs of the Taunton area and to the special needs of each client.

To confront these difficulties, the traditional hierarchical structure was replaced by a matrix organization that is capable of focusing its resources simultaneously on providing geographic services and fulfilling organizational functions. The matrix structure illustrated in Figure 10.1 was designed specifically to respond to (a) dual-focused outside pressure, (b) the need for high information-processing capacity, and (c) the necessity of sharing resources.[4]

EVALUATION

Three independent dimensions of change were chosen for evaluation: political response, changes in effects and in the cost of services to client groups, and bureaucratic change, including personnel changes and organizational changes.

A *political response* follows most political initiatives in the field of health care. It may be positive or negative and may vary in intensity. It may come from taxpayers and their representatives who are dissatisfied

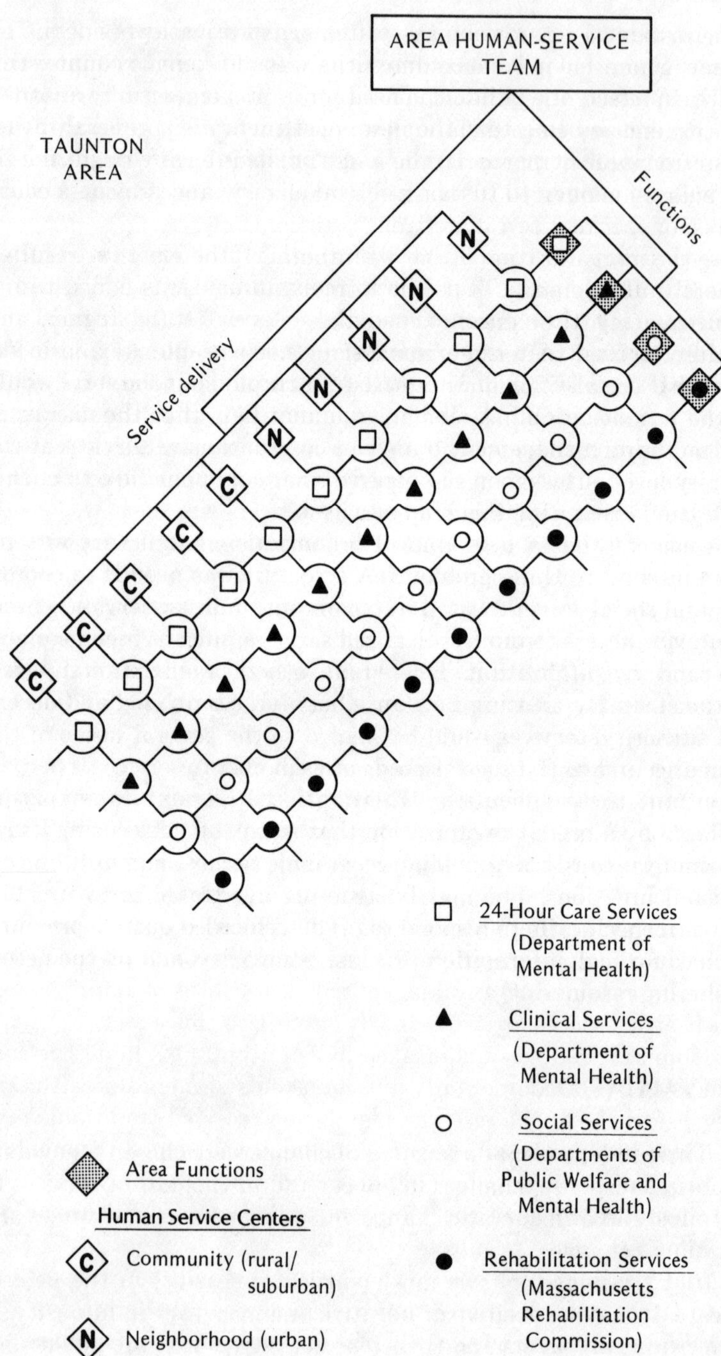

Figure 10.1. Area-based human-service matrix organization.

with the results of a new delivery system or from employees of the bureaucracy whose environments have changed. Frequently many concerns are expressed other than the need for improvement in care and/or a reduction in costs. Because human services are funded primarily by tax revenues from which appropriations must be made each year during the legislative session devoted to the state's budgetary process, a positive political response is required if a change is to continue.

Before the reorganization of the Taunton area, the state cared for approximately 400 mentally ill people from Taunton each year. The only available treatment consisted of custodial services located at the Taunton State Hospital. After reorganization, 4,000 people were provided with either hospital- or community-based social and clinical services. Because the number of admissions and the duration of confinements decreased so sharply, there was no increase in inflation-adjusted costs.

The response to this change is apparent on many political levels. Individual commitment to the human-service centers was measured by the contribution of thousands of volunteer hours. Community support was demonstrated by the willingness of towns to contribute local tax revenue to maintain the centers. Employee support was indicated by the 52 staff members who moved from hospital roles to community-based services. Another measure of political success relates to the fact that many basic ideas from Taunton are becoming building blocks for changing the state human-service system.

Change occurring in the *cost effectiveness* of human services is perhaps the most critical dimension of evaluation. What benefit does intervention confer on the people who receive the service? At what cost? Which group of interventions makes the best use of scarce resources?

Mental health and human services are plagued by the lack of critical standards for evaluating effectiveness. The general posture reflects the belief that medical care is effective. The belief creates a placebo effect that permits considering any kind of care the cause of improvement. Mental-health services are particularly subject to this effect.

A randomized trial was undertaken in Taunton to evaluate the costs and effects of two fundamentally different kinds of mental-health services.[5] One segment of the research population received traditional services provided by clinicians. The other segment was helped through volunteer problem-solving teams, a resource developed from one of the central theoretical ideas of the Taunton reorganization—the use of low-cost, community-based resources.

The trial was set up to ensure that patients would be randomly assigned to either a single, state-employed, professional therapist or to a team of local volunteers who would provide counseling and support and would share practical experiences.

The trial showed that both groups of clients improved. The difference was significant at the .01 level. Some measurements of outcome showed no difference between the results obtained by teams and those obtained by professionals, whereas others indicated that professional therapists did a better job. To some extent, this study demonstrated that clinicians and volunteers were equally able to deliver effective services. However, the status of the provider subjects the state to different costs. A salaried clinician costs the government more than what it pays for the services of a volunteer. Actual delivery costs for clinical services are approximately double those of volunteer problem-solving teams. If we assume that the clinicians did better, a 40 percent improvement on one of five instruments is achieved at an additional marginal cost of $151 per client.

Bureaucratic evaluation can also occur on a number of levels. Two were selected to evaluate Taunton: personnel changes and changes in the organization. Employees at many different levels left institutional roles that were rigidly fixed in the hospital hierarchy to assume new community-based jobs. On the whole, these employees responded positively to the new activities and brought revitalized energy and resources to work at no extra cost to the state.[6]

Workers who object to a change can block it for decades, either from the top of or from within the structure. They may allow change to occur on paper but not in practice. Students of bureaucracy have studied this phenomenon for a long time. The reactionary attitude of bureaucrats is one reason why the good name that Max Weber gave bureaucracy has become a derogatory term.

As we have noted, the union agreed to the change after its members became convinced of the benefits. However, despite considerable efforts in Taunton, little change occurred in the civil service. Consequently, it became necessary to circumvent the intent of the civil service.

The complete human-service matrix organization was never realized. The community human-service centers were operational for mental-health clients and the users of many other local programs. Welfare social services and rehabilitation services, although located at the centers for a period of time, never became part of integrated service delivery.

Success was achieved with the differentiation of the mental-health organization into two geographic levels. Twenty-four-hour care and clinical functions were centralized at the area level, whereas the delivery of services was decentralized to 10 communities and neighborhoods.

Because of its innovations, Taunton was able to attract skilled professionals who had previously preferred to work elsewhere. However, it is ironical to note that so many professionals became available that they tended to drive the volunteer teams out of existence.

HUMAN SERVICES AND THE STATE OF MASSACHUSETTS

The Human-Service Environment

The changes in the Taunton area from 1970 to 1976 occurred in relative isolation from the rest of the state, where decentralization stopped at the area level. We will now consider human services in the state of Massachusetts, and to do so we must begin with the federal bureaucratic structure.

The primary agency responsible for human services at the national level is the Department of Health, Education and Welfare (HEW). HEW is composed of hundreds of categorical agencies overseeing programs in income maintenance, health, general education, special education, mental health, social services, and rehabilitation. Other federal departments that are independent of HEW control community development, employment, housing, and corrections.

Each HEW agency has counterparts in the fifty states. The state agencies are partially funded and regulated by the federal agencies (each agency has a different funding formula and different regulations) and partially funded by state revenues. A federal department that is organized on the basis of categorical agencies puts heavy pressure on states seeking federal funds to organize categorically. In return, the states pay the price implicit in the lack of coordination that prevents organizations from delivering cost-effective services in an area. Half of the states lack the executive capacity, for example, systems managers corresponding to the secretary of HEW, to coordinate human services within the states. In the absence of a human-services cabinet, each subagency in a state exercises considerable independence.

Every one of the fifty states has a different approach to service delivery. In addition, each agency within a state defines in a unique way the structure and the process of service delivery. Categorical organization has led to uncontrollable increases in expenditures and hundreds of uncoordinated field offices in each state. There were 240 uncoordinated field offices in Massachusetts at the beginning of 1977.

The current central organization of human services in Massachusetts is shown in Figure 10.2. As can be seen, Massachusetts has an Executive Office of Human Services that reviews agency activities and performs some coordinating functions among agencies.

The Role of Theory

The overall characteristics of a human-service delivery system can be described by 10 variables. These variables are summarized in Table 10.3.

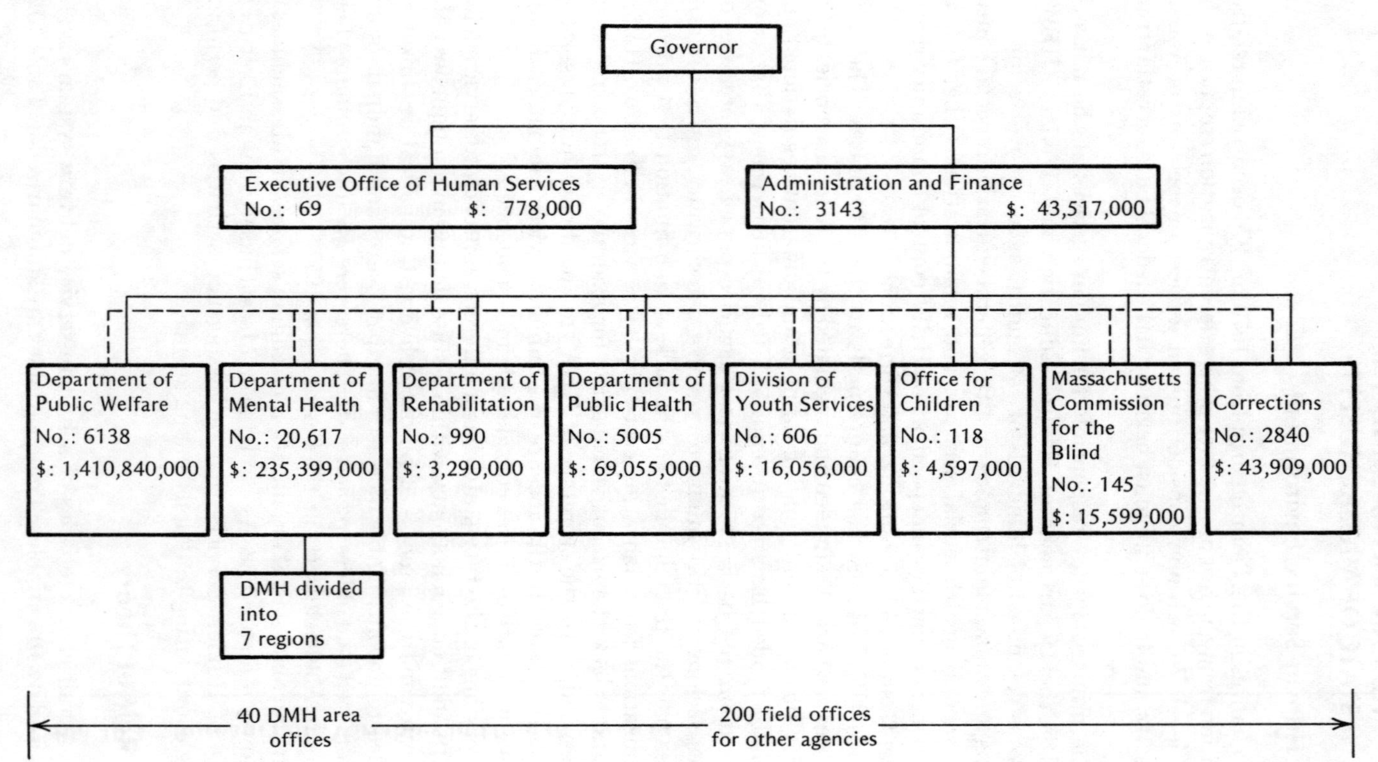

Figure 10.2. Massachusetts Central Agency structure with 1977 expenses and number of positions.

Table 10.3 Bureaucratic Variables in Human Services

Variable Name	*Definition*[a]	*End Points*[b]
1. Level of government	*Responsibility for providing each kind of service may be held by state or local government or both.* For example, local (county) government in Florida provides EMERGENCY food, housing, and income transfers, whereas state government provides LONG-TERM food, housing, and income transfers.	Local government/state government.
2. Economic approach	*Delivery system may operate as a market place* (in which agencies compete for resources and clients shop for services) *or as a single-entry system* (in which client gains access to services at one location and negotiates for the best fit between the problem and available public services). Historically, the United States' economic approach has been based on free enterprise in the market place and has assumed continual expansion of resources and services. Some human services cannot be effectively delivered in this context.	Public/Private
3. Spending approach	*Organizational change may result from new spending* (which represents overall expansion) *or from spending reallocated from one service to another.*	Reallocation/expansion
4. Organizational structure	At the central and area levels, *each categorical agency may exist independently or may be subordinated to a*	Human service/categorical

Table 10.3 *(continued)*

Variable Name	*Definition*[a]	*End Points*[b]
	larger whole through a human service structure; the human service structure may be either coordinated or integrated.	
5. Level of authority	*Budget and personnel decisions may be made in central offices or in the field offices* where service delivery occurs.	Decentralized/centralized
6. Organizational roles	*Management and service delivery may be performed by specialists* (trained in a particular discipline) *or generalists* (skilled in analyzing situations as a whole and in affecting the interactions of their components, which may include use of specialist resources).	Generalist/specialist
7. *Service delivery structure*	*Delivery system may be structured as a network* (with varying numbers of formal and informal relationships at critical activity points) *or it may have no connecting structures* (agencies operate without communication or coordination). At the present time, independent agencies consist of: *human service* agencies, providing health education income transfers	Network/independent agencies

Table 10.3 (*continued*)

Variable Name	*Definition*[a]	*End Points*[b]
	housing employment social services mental health welfare social services rehabilitation children and youth services elderly services family services retardation (mostly OHDS- and NIMH-supported) Note multiple duplications, evidence of the current critical problems in administering services effectively.	
8. *Community*	*The state organization can relate* its political, bureaucratic, and service delivery activities *to different kinds of communities,* e.g., geographic community or communities of interest. Each kind of community provides a different kind and number of resources, a different sense of "belonging" for its members.	Geographic community/community of interest
9. *Service approach*	*Two kinds of human services have been defined, and approaches to providing them should vary accordingly.*	Inseparable service/separable service

Table 10.3 (*continued*)

Variable Name	*Definition*[a]	*End Points*[b]
	SEPARABLE services occur in clearly defined units/products, have a beginning and an end, and are quantifiable. Examples: income, housing, food, medication, surgery, psychological testing. Change occurs in the client irrespective of government action when the intervention is complete. INSEPARABLE services involve a process in which change depends on modifying interactions among forces and on the expert judgment of service providers. Separable services are generally delivered to individuals for specific reasons. Inseparable services involve networks of people who interact with each other, with the intention of changing their ongoing relationships.	
10. *Client approach*	*A "client" can be defined as an individual or a social network*. The area of focus for an individual may be a particular problem or the "whole" person. The area of focus for a social network is a particular group of actors and the relationships among them. (See service approach above.)	Social network/individual client

[a] This analysis is based on a "service by geography" organization. Some definitions would change for a "function by geography" organization.

[b] The end-point labels should convey the present thinking in human services: Each end has a zero-sum value, presently dominated by the right-hand value of each variable.

The current system in Massachusetts is heavily oriented toward the right-hand value for each variable presented in the figure. Massachusetts state government has historically emphasized state control, a marketplace approach to services, expansion, categorical services, centralized decision making, predominance of specialists, independent agencies, communities of special interest, separable services, and treatment of individual clients.

The development of human-service organizations in Massachusetts requires a shift in emphasis on each variable from the right, which dominates current activities, to the left. It is important that the shift not be a *replacement* of one value by the other but reflect the establishment of flexible organizational mechanisms that allow responses contingent on the best fit for any given situation.

Managing the Change

In 1975 the third secretary of the Executive Office of Human Services was appointed by the governor. He recognized that hundreds of field offices were unrelated to each other, allowing the duplication of services. He also observed that within what was essentially a fixed budget, interest groups were relentless in their demand for and manipulation of funds. Each professional group seemed to define its area of focus as the most important facet of human services. Three hundred fifty-one cities and towns, crippled by rising property taxes, all took different positions toward being partners in the overall human-service system. Most challenging of all was the fact that authority over budget and personnel assignment resided in the Executive Office of Administration and Finance and within the human-services agencies.

It was clear that the Massachusetts electorate, like the nation as a whole, demanded that government not expand further until it had (1) broadened the base of services and (2) improved their quality. Change, therefore, would no longer be dependent on new funding. Fortunately, considerable public resources that were being spent on human services could become part of an attempt to improve the overall system.

In October 1976 the secretary of human services produced a policy memorandum entitled Area Strategy.[7] It proposed five major responses to existing problems. First was the establishment of 40 management teams consisting of the agency directors in each area. The second called for increased decentralization of authority to these teams. The third proposed increased budget flexibility at this decentralized level within a philosophy of cost containment. The fourth recognized the education bureaucracy—an independent cabinet—as a critical actor in the executive reorganization. The fifth emphasized reform from the "bottom up," that is, events in the service-delivery system would become critical sources of information for effecting overall system change. In the last two years extensive efforts have been undertaken to implement this policy.

The political position of this statewide experiment is subject to change from a number of directions. The legislature could impose a change in direction affecting area strategy. There will be a new secretary of the Executive Office of Human Services and a new governor who may or may not promote these changes.

CONCLUSION

In the early 1970s a confluence of unique environmental conditions made possible the move to community human-service centers in Taunton. Some of the theoretical concepts applied during this transition included: deinstitutionalization, social networks, community development, problem-solving teams, and matrix organization. The change was managed in spite of a lack of external funding. Evaluation occurred in terms of political response, cost-effectiveness of services, and bureaucratic change.

The ideas initially tested in Taunton helped promote change at the state level. Area strategy was developed as a way of improving the state bureaucracy without incurring new expenditures. Change in the overall organization, as proposed by the 10 variables, could be achieved through the development of 40 area-based delivery systems created within the existing structure.

NOTES

1. A discussion of the movement of these resources is contained in W. Robert Curtis, "From State Hospital to Integrated Human Service System," *Health Care Management Review,* vol. 1, no. 2 (Spring 1976), and in Julia Herskowitz and W. Robert Curtis, "The Psychiatric Hospital Employee: A Resource for Social Change," *Health Care Management Review,* vol. 2, no. 1 (Winter 1977).
2. For a more detailed analysis of this intervention, see W. Robert Curtis, "Community Human Service Networks: New Roles for Mental Health Workers," *Psychiatric Annals,* vol. 3, no. 7 (July 1973), and W. Robert Curtis, "Team Problems Solving in a Social Network," *Psychiatric Annals,* vol. 4, no. 12 (December 1974).
3. The various aspects of this problem are analyzed in W. Robert Curtis and Duncan Neuhauser, "Providing Specialized Coordinated Human Services to Communities: The Organizational Problem and a Potential Solution," Position Paper no. 4, *Ford Foundation Seminar on the Delivery of Urban Health Services,* Harvard School of Public Health.

4. See Stanley Davis and Paul Lawrence, *Matrix* (Reading, Mass.: Addison-Wesley Publishing Company, 1977), and W. Robert Curtis, "What Follows Services Integration? Simulated Decentralized State Organizations Delivering Comprehensive Human Services" (Social Matrix Research, Inc., 1977).
5. W. Robert Curtis, "The Clinical Trial: A Study of Social Network and Clinical Intervention," Ph. D. Dissertation, Harvard School of Public Health, Boston, Mass., 1978.
6. Julia Herskowitz and W. Robert Curtis reviewed the various effects of deinstitutionalization on state hospital staff. Topics such as resource reallocation, employee reactions, training, retraining, and staffing patterns were discussed in detail. See "Deinstitutionalization and Its Effects on Employees," *Social Matrix Research Monograph Publication Series,* Boston, Mass., 1977.
7. For five publications that present a policy framework as well as an implementation plan and were designed to present overviews and analyses of organization tensions, see W. Robert Curtis, "Area Strategy," *Social Matrix Research Publications Series,* Boston, Mass., 1978.

Chapter 11

Toward Coordination of Health and Social Services: Substance and Means in Cooperation

Ragnar Berfenstam and Ragnhild Placht

THE HOLISTIC VIEW OF MAN AS A PRINCIPLE IN COMMUNITY SERVICE

In recent years there has been a lively debate in many countries concerning ways of making social welfare and health services more effective as well as more humane and more oriented toward prevention. This debate has also taken place in Sweden.

A modern idea that has increasingly gained acceptance in Sweden is the holistic view. It is founded on the increasing realization that close links exist between medical and social circumstances. In practice, the holistic view suggests that those who work with people in need of help seek to consider simultaneously the physical, psychological, and social needs of individuals. It also follows that one works toward coordination of social and medical services in order to use the resources of society to help individuals.

WEAKNESSES RESULTING FROM A LACK OF COORDINATION

Swedish officials, through a number of official statements, have announced guidelines for coordinating community services. Coordination is considered necessary because of increasing specialization.[1,2] Social and health services are performed under the auspices of municipalities and county councils, respectively. Statutes delineate the areas for which the respective bodies are responsible. The two bodies have established separate systems for financing. The education of personnel is carried out independently. Increased specialization within the health and social services has also sharpened differences between the respective professional groups. Working in social and medical services often confers different degrees of prestige and status.

The consequences of differential development are many. The patient/client has sometimes been caught between the two services. Lacking comprehensive analysis, the risk of losing essential background information exists. Such losses result in the dispensation of inadequate help. Time is lost when the patient/client is shifted between different professionals. There are great risks of duplicating work and suboptimal returns.

COORDINATION—A NEW DEAL

An increasing number of groups have been arguing for the necessity of coordination. The idea can easily be traced to political debates. Coordination is relatively well advanced if one considers the official attitude toward the need to coordinate medical and social services. Within a number of higher administrative bodies, a common view of community health and welfare services has been adopted. In recent years this view has influenced broad planning principles, for example, those concerning the care of and the responsibility for children with social or physical handicaps and support for youth. Coordinating these programs involves schools, police, and recreational centers. This view has also gained acceptance among groups that provide care and services for the old. Joint committees have been created at local levels in order to improve care provided for the aged and chronically ill, and these measures have effected certain economic gains.

In recent years another principle has been articulated. It involves expanding the orientation of coordinated activities from the individual to groups and communities. The expansion of coordinated activities may contribute toward making general preventive endeavors more broadly based and may assist in achieving greater penetration derived from the use of practical social and medical knowledge.

A DEFINITION OF CONCEPTS

Some terms are used interchangeably in the literature on interdisciplinary cooperation in primary care to describe various forms of relationships between medical and social work performed at different organizational and administrative levels. Usually no distinction is made between such concepts as cooperation, collaboration, coordination, integration, and team work. How these concepts are defined depends in part on prevalent organizational structures. For the purpose of this article, the following basic definitions are used.

Co-operation, according to *The Advanced Learner's Dictionary of Current English,* means "working together toward a common purpose," and in this context, the word is often used to describe different arrangements of cooperative efforts undertaken at the field level between medical and social personnel.

Collaboration appears to be a more general term, for it is defined simply as "working together."

Integration, on the other hand, is defined as "combining into a whole." It seems therefore to have a more pronounced organizational meaning. Medical social workers, for example, may be regarded as integrated into the medical-service system in several countries, including Sweden.

Coordination means "to bring or put into proper relation." It can thus be considered a loose form of integration. Therefore, coordination may be an adequate term to cover different organizational and administrative efforts that *facilitate* cooperation between medical and social personnel. Coordination may be introduced when a formally-integrated system is neither desirable nor feasible.

Team, in the context of health and social services, should be reserved for a relatively small group of people, the nucleus of which is comprised of a doctor, a nurse, and a social worker. This denotation underlines the interdisciplinary aspect of the concept. The concept sometimes connotes different meanings. In England, for example, only cooperation that obtains between doctors and nurses has been defined as team work. (1) Used in this way, team work is a synonym for interdisciplinary cooperation, albeit the latter term is more general and vague. In this article, for the purpose of clarification, we call teams sociomedical teams.

We hope that these definitions are adequate. Although we would like to stress the importance of drawing distinctions between these concepts, national differences in organizational structures make the formulation of precise definitions a difficult task.

TO WHAT EXTENT HAS SWEDEN ACHIEVED PRACTICAL COORDINATION OF COMMUNITY SERVICES?

Coordination demands the reorganization of health and social services at every stage of delivery as well as changes in attitudes. Consequently, in order to effect coordination between medical and social services in Sweden, the central administration was reorganized. At first the ministries for medical and social affairs were merged into one ministry (the Ministry for Social and Medical Affairs), and then, in 1968, the Board of Social Welfare and the Board of Health merged to become the Board of Health and Welfare.

As far as coordination aimed at joint planning with respect to health and welfare is concerned, efforts have been intensified at the levels below the national administration. However, planning has sometimes been conducted in a vague and superficial way.[3]

The National Board of Health and Welfare is engaged in a number of programs involving coordinating activities in the field of health and social services, that is, the areas for which the county councils and the municipalities are responsible. These programs differ with respect to goals and organizational designs. On the whole, three different organizational models are being tested.

The *first* model is based on the assumption that cooperation occurs only in a limited number of very serious cases that impel ad hoc groups to examine cases thoroughly and devise plans that deal with every aspect of welfare and further care. The core members of the group are the doctor and the social worker, but representatives of other community bodies participate when there is reason to do so. The aim is the coordination of efforts with respect to the realistic formulation of goals and the realization of objectives.

The *second* model suggests the movement of a social worker into a medical setting and his or her subsequent integration into a medical setting, which is facilitated by working with a doctor or doctors in cases that come to the health center. A variation of this model suggests that when a doctor is placed in a locality that provides social welfare, he or she becomes involved in the analysis and treatment of serious, multiproblem cases. In a number of large towns in Sweden, one can find this kind of doctor. He or she is known as the social-medical officer.

The *third* model suggests coordination with respect to location and organization. Accordingly, one devises a plan to encourage cooperation in order to ameliorate the patient's/client's problems in the best possible way. The geographic catchment areas are the same for both medical and social services. Both services may even have offices in the same building.

DIFFICULTIES—OBSTACLES TO COORDINATION AND COOPERATION

In Sweden, experimental and investigative work is continuing in order to obtain more knowledge about how coordination functions. A number of project spokesmen have reported their experiences. The National Board of Health and Welfare collated these reports in order to present a collective picture of the experiences of ongoing activities.[4] The purpose of this compilation is to give guidance to those who intend to coordinate social and medical services at the local level. These reports, however, are not based on systematic study. No efforts have been made to distinguish between difficulties of an organizational nature (coordination) and difficulties emanating from the actual team-work situation (cooperation). Changes made in a number of places in Sweden differ, as was mentioned earlier, both with respect to goals and organizational design. Furthermore, no sharp distinction is made between goals and means. This circumstance, together with deficiencies in the general design of programs, complicates evaluation.

As a rule, however, there have been no difficulties in effecting plans that are of a strictly organizational nature. In general, politicians and officials at regional and local organizational and administrative levels seem to agree that coordinating activities in the field of health and social services is justified. This much can be said. The changes that have been made involve no profound or far-reaching interference in the exercise of the duties of those who are affected, including politicians and officials at regional, local, and administrative levels and professionals who are directly involved in team work.

For the latter group, the important question is whether the holistic view is accepted and has actually resulted in a changed way of working. Lack of knowledge prevents us from answering this question. Studies concerning cooperation in teams, conducted in Sweden and abroad, concentrated on factors that render difficult the analysis of interdisciplinary cooperation. Circumstances that were reported to worsen interdisciplinary cooperation include difficulties emanating from trying to bridge the gap between a system of knowledge that is based on natural science and a system that is humanistic. This gap results in a lack of appropriate working methods and frustrations arising from changed professional roles. Differences in status and attitude among team members who lack the experience of working in a group and of making joint decisions are only a few of the difficulties involved in team work.[5,6]

The crucial question is whether interdisciplinary cooperation based on the holistic view has exerted any kind of impact on patients/clients. No studies of significance have to our knowledge been devoted to such an objective. Irrespective of the immense technical and methodological difficulties that one would encounter in studying such an enterprise, there is every reason to intensify such efforts. In Sweden the time does not yet seem ripe for evaluating effects.

COOPERATION IN PRACTICE

Cooperation in the field may be carried out and is often done so on an informal and unplanned basis. Those who have responsibility for the patient/client make contact with one another to analyze and solve an individual case that is believed to be susceptible to cooperative endeavors.

The methods and the nature of cooperation vary considerably. Consequently, formal cooperation may include regularly-held conferences and actual team work performed by medical and social personnel. Evaluating all these forms of cooperation would be difficult to carry out.

Cooperation can be made easier if joint education programs are arranged. One can thus achieve a reciprocal appreciation of the principles of cooperation as well as teach suitable working methods.

Those who wish to work in this area should realize that cooperation is complicated, that it demands an ongoing in-service education in order to increase knowledge, that it presupposes a change of attitude, and that the participants need to agree on a new way of working to achieve a common objective. Such efforts usually take time. When obstacles arise, problems need to be tackled at all relevant levels, that is, by both local boards and professional categories.

HOW CAN COORDINATION BE SUCCESSFUL?

Planning for the future has not been hindered by the difficulties and obstacles that have been reported by those engaged in such work.

The responsible national bodies maintain that coordination should be the aim. A memorandum from the National Board of Health and Welfare in 1975 emphasized that coordination should not be limited to the health, welfare, and school services involved in a joint health program.[7] Others should also be included, for example, vocational-training, rehabilitation, local health-insurance, and social-security officers.

The importance of formulating a common plan and achieving a common objective was emphasized in this memorandum, which also stressed the importance of locating the services in the same building and of drawing boundaries demarcating the jurisdictions in which the geographical service areas of the various branches of the services would operate. Coterminality is supposed to ensure that the services share responsibility for the same population. These guidelines, needless to say, were designed to facilitate effective team work and the efficient use of available resources.

THE TIERP PROJECT AS AN EXAMPLE OF COORDINATED PROGRAMS

We will mention some of the findings derived from research carried out by the Department of Social Medicine in Uppsala with respect to the coordination of services in the Tierp area. This work relates to the concept of coordination defined by the third model mentioned above. Over a period of three years, practical experience has been gained from this project. The participants include the Tierp Municipality that is responsible for social welfare, including the home-help service and the school health service, and the Uppsala County Council that is responsible for all kinds of health services within the area.[8]

The area, which is mainly rural, is centered on Tierp, a town of about 4,000 inhabitants. Including a number of smaller villages and settlements, the population totals about 21,000 inhabitants. In Tierp itself is a joint health center shared by medical and social services. There are a number of common facilities, including a cafeteria and a common room where all personnel groups usually meet at least once a week. The municipality is divided into five districts, the boundaries of which are common to the three major services: public health and medical care, social and welfare care, and schools. In other words, there is a common subdivision that forms five efficient working units for the three separate services.

From the beginning of the project, the parties involved, that is, the National Board of Health and Welfare, the Uppsala County Council, and the Tierp Municipality, agreed on joint action based on the holistic view, that is, the close relationship between an individual and his or her environment, taking medical and social factors into consideration. The principles were enunciated in an "approach report" aimed at coordinating efforts at all levels in the municipality, that is, the political, administrative, and field levels (see Figure 11.1). As the figure shows, the organizational structure devised to ensure the success of the project includes, first, a political steering group called the coordinating committee; sec-

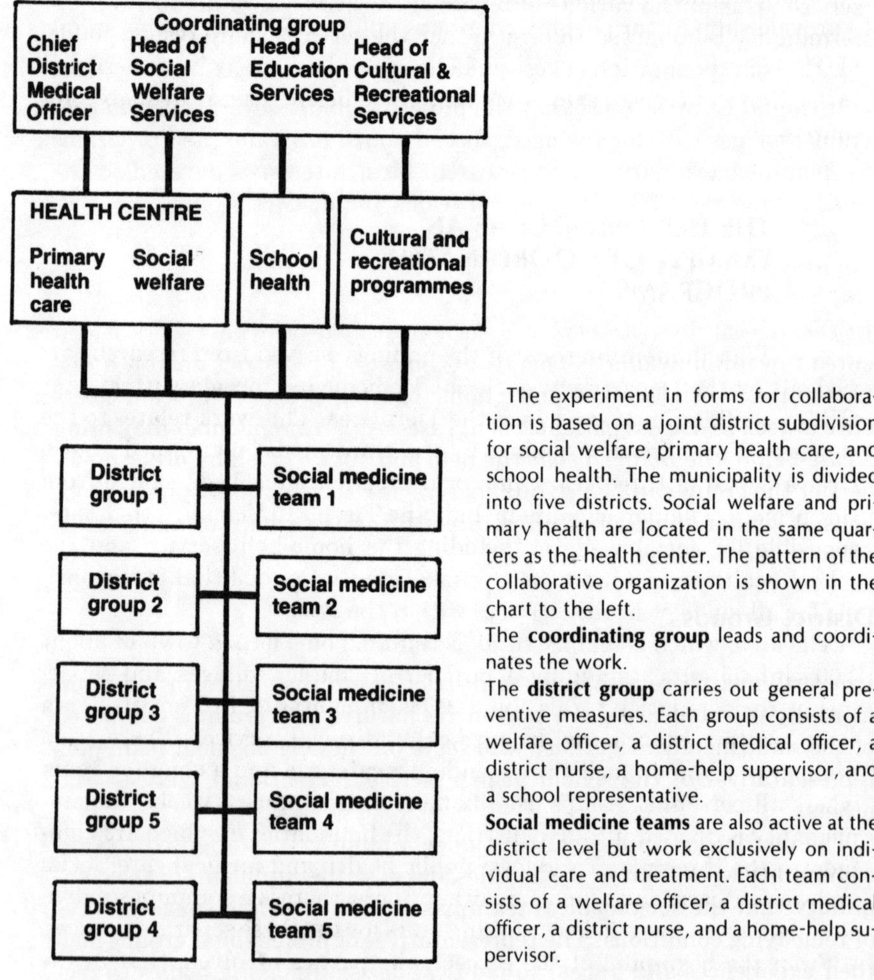

Figure 11.1. The collaborative organization.

ond, a coordination group comprised of the head administrators for health, social welfare, schools, and recreational services; and, third, two field groups, called district groups and sociomedical teams, for every district within the municipality.

At all levels joint action is directed toward the achievement of three equally important objectives:

to ensure that the local districts within the municipality form an efficient unit and function satisfactorily;
to reduce the need for social welfare, primary health care, and school health by achieving good conditions in the area;
to provide support for people and groups afflicted by ill health or social problems.

It should be mentioned that the project includes several specific programs, such as care for the aged, special youth programs, and programs for planning, evaluation, and research. Most interest is devoted to the joint field work of the sociomedical teams and district groups.

Sociomedical Teams

In every local district there is a sociomedical team whose work is oriented toward individuals. This team consists of a district doctor, a district nurse, a social worker, and a home-help supervisor. The team meets once a week to discuss patient/client cases. Any team member may bring a case before the team so that the help and advice given by other members of the group can be used to analyze and solve an individual's problems. A similar approach is often directed toward groups of individuals, for example, families.

District Groups

In every area there also exists a district group that performs environmentally-oriented tasks of a preventive nature. This group is composed of the same members as those who serve on the sociomedical team plus representatives of the school health service, recreational services, and others.

The district group meets about once a month. It is oriented toward community work, that is, it identifies and describes problems in the community that the sociomedical team has encountered and suggests ways of remedying conditions. The representatives of professional groups pool their experiences and appeal to political decision-making bodies to rectify deficiencies. Such problems may derive from housing deficiencies, environments harmful to children and youth, dangerous traffic conditions, the lack of playgounds for young children as well as occupational therapy and entertainments for the elderly.

The members of the district group find their work stimulating as well as difficult. It requires knowledge and experience of community work to be able to understand and deal with indigenous problems. The members find it difficult to apprehend the scope of their powers because, in spite of the guidelines under which they function, they are an informal group. In general, however, a positive attitude prevails among group members toward community-oriented tasks.

Sociomedical Field Work in Teams

We have concentrated our interest on the efforts of the sociomedical teams, that is, on how people from different professions learn to work together and on the content of such cooperative work. The district doctor, the district nurse, the social worker, and the home-help supervisor were interviewed in 1974, before the project started, and then one year after cooperation had begun. The objective was to try to assess how professional people felt toward one another as well as how they felt about not having been especially trained and not having worked together before the project was initiated.

The result of analyzing one year's cooperative efforts demonstrated that all professional groups affirmed the efficacy of cooperation based on the concept of the team.[9] Several expressed the opinion that the method used to discuss patients and clients was of great importance. It was also pointed out that meeting as a team facilitates ad hoc contacts in special and sometimes urgent cases because team members know one another and each member's area of competence as well as his or her way of approaching problems. Of course, there are always people in such a group who doubt whether team work is worthwhile, considering the time consumed by this kind of work and the sometimes limited help that can be given to solve individual patient/client problems.

The interview also produced quantitative information that was used to estimate the number of contacts between members of the teams outside team conferences. The analysis showed that there were many such contacts every month. There were, for example, many contacts not only between doctors and district nurses in dealing with health problems but also between doctors and social workers in the municipality regarding both diagnostic and therapeutic work. Of course, the frequency of the contacts, which varied greatly, depended to a great extent on personal opinions and attitudes.

WHAT IS THE CONTENT OF TEAM WORK?

An evaluation team work, such as that described, should ascertain as its ultimate goal whether the patient—the client—received more adequate help through team work than he or she would have received through the more traditional way of handling individual problems. Because this goal is too difficult to attain, we concentrated on the content of the work performed in the teams, how the work was performed, what obstacles intervened in team work, and what factors favor effective team work.

Four different teams were studied by a participant observer for a period of approximately seven months during 1976–1977. The observer did not actively take part in the discussions of patients/clients. Instead, detailed notes were taken during the meetings. Some of the meetings were tape-recorded in order to establish a control against which to evaluate the reliability of the method of note taking. The data base for this study consisted of the computation of certain variables, for example, the number of team meetings, the number of team members present, the number of cases that were considered by each team, the activity entered into by team members during the discussions.

During the observational period, three of the four teams met regularly about once a week. The fourth team met only a few times. Not all professionals were represented at every meeting. Nonattendance, however, was the result of leaves of absence. Activity on the part of team members was measured in two ways. Regarding the number of contributions made during the discussions, there were no differences among professional groups. However, with respect to the number of cases that were brought up for discussion by team members, social workers and home-help supervisors initiated the discussion of about twice as many cases as did doctors and nurses.

The total number of cases that were subjected to discussions in the four teams were 277, 180, 348, and 19, respectively. The average number of cases that were discussed per meeting were 13, 9, 11, and 6.

The cooperative efforts of these four teams concerned approximately 4 percent of households in the teams' service areas.

When consideration is given to the fact that the discussions often involved the same households, the total number of cases dropped to 81, 96, 128, and 16, respectively. In other words, the four teams discussed each household, on the average, 3.4, 1.9, 2.9, and 1.2 times, respectively.

Some of the findings invite speculation. For example, why were the cases discussed so few times? Are problems usually so trivial that they warrant little discussion, or are there difficulties in effecting cooperation? These and similar questions will be subjected to a deeper analysis.

Other findings from this study relate to attempts to judge the value of team work. Cooperation that was apparent in a sample of 30 cases (discussions concerning 30 households) was subjected to a closer study. The observer's detailed notes were compiled and were presented to a panel of experts. The panel, whose members had no knowledge of or connection with the area under study, was composed of experienced officials from the same professional groups as those in the teams. The members of the panel were instructed to assess aspects of a formal nature with respect to case work *and* the benefit of working as a team. The panel was also instructed to assess cooperation in the 30 cases by analyzing 8 aspects of team work that can be considered basic requirements in the handling of a case:

1. Problem formulation: How well was each problem formulated?
2. Background information: To what extent was the necessary background information provided?
3. The thoroughness of each discussion.
4. The purposefulness of each discussion.
5. Comprehensiveness of judgment: To what extent was the assessment of the patient/client based on the holistic view?
6. Comprehensiveness in planning: To what extent was due attention paid to all the patient's/client's needs in planning rehabilitation?
7. Appropriateness of the choice of treatment.
8. Follow-up: To what extent were follow-ups planned and regular?

The handling of a case was assessed according to a predetermined scale that contained criteria for ranking how well each basic requirement had been met. A scale, ranging from 0–3, was provided. The better the performance, the higher the rank. The system of point setting, which was solely constructed for the use of the panel, is explained in detail in a manual.

Some of the basic requirements were also used to evaluate the benefit that may accrue to a team in casework. A different scale was devised for this purpose, although the same range—0–3—was retained.

Conducting two analyses enabled us to separate the quality of the handling of cases from judgments concerning the benefit of working as a team. The reason for conducting separate analyses was based on the belief that good performance does not necessarily mean good team work.

Consequently, the panel's rankings relate both to how well the teams handled their cases and to the degree to which working as a team contributed to that effect. The judgments made by the panel are undergoing analysis. We are very much aware of the fact that the work done by the teams has only been judged by *one* panel whose members displayed variations in judgment. We are also aware of the fact that only two aspects of the teams' work were judged and that these limitations impinge on the findings.

Some preliminary findings, however, indicate that improvements can be made in fulfilling the eight basic requirements. Improvements can be made in the handling of cases and in increasing the benefits that can be derived from working as a team. The findings also show that there were consistent and relatively great variations among the teams.

The cooperation manifest in the teams under study is not of an optimal nature, according to the judgments made by the panel of experts. The professionals in the teams had no prior training in team work. Their existing work load appears to be heavy, and their willingness to be observed and evaluated must therefore be greatly admired.

We are going to concentrate our efforts on giving the team members feedback, that is, present to them the findings of this study. Seminars on the methodology of teamwork will also be arranged. At these seminars considerable attention will be paid to the formal aspects of a team meeting. These aspects will be based on the panel's judgments regarding the basic requirements. This feedback will provide an opportunity for improving the work of the teams.

CONCLUDING REMARKS

After four years, those who have been engaged in cooperative work were asked whether this work should continue in the absence of encouragement from the project's directors. The answers were positive. Many have experienced feelings of "belonging together," of solidarity, and of unity. For example, in recurring problems of a sociomedical nature that require great imagination and thoroughness to diagnose and treat and involve great risks of failure, working in teams may give members security, satisfaction, and assurance because responsibility is shared. These gains certainly justify extra expenditures of time. The respondents emphasized that finding solutions to problems confronted in day-to-day casework was much easier when one knew the other members of the team.

In the model that we have described, representatives of professions working in health and social services were not trained for this kind of cooperative work. Therefore, time had to elapse before cooperation could be achieved. Preliminary findings indicate that methodological problems are crucial. We are of the opinion that much more must be done to provide basic and continuous training of professional groups before we can form teams that will be effective. Perhaps common training at the undergraduate level, consisting of joint seminars and discussions as well as training in team work, will have to be provided before we can attain this goal: to achieve such a high degree of cooperation that we can realistically speak of applying the holistic view in an effort to confront the patient's/client's problems and needs and to improve the kinds of assistance that we can render to him or her.

REFERENCES

1. Gilmore, M., Bruce, N., and Hunt, M. *The Work of the Nursing Team in General Practice.* Council for the Education and Training of Health Visitors. London, 1974.
2. Kohn, R. "Coordination of Health and Welfare Services in Four Countries: Austria, Italy, Poland, and Sweden." *Public Health in Europe* (6). Regional Office for Europe WHO. Copenhagen, 1977.
3. Landstingsförbundet, Svenska Kommunförbundet, Socialstyrelsen och Spri: *Primärvård Äldreomsorger Samverkan.* Stockholm, 1977.
4. Socialstyrelsen. *Samarbete mellan socialvård samt hälsooch sjukvård.* Stockholm, 1977.
5. Banta, R. F., and Fox, R. C. "Role Strains of a Health Care Team in a Poverty Community." *Soc. Sci. & Med.* (1972) 6: 697–722.
6. Rubin, I. M., and Beckhard, R. "Factors Influencing the Effectiveness of Health Teams." *Milbank Mem. Fund Q.* (1972) 50: 317–335, Part 1.
7. The National Swedish Board of Health and Welfare. *The Swedish Health Services in the 1980s.* Stockholm, 1976.
8. The National Board of Health and Welfare. The Tierp Project—Its Objectives, Organization, and Fields of Activity. Stockholm, 1977.
9. Berfenstam, R., and Smedby, B. "Samverkan mellan medicinsk och social vård." *Socialmedicinsk tidskrift* (1976) 53: 365–372.

Chapter 12

Priorities in the English National Health Service

R. G. S. Brown

INTRODUCTION

The innovation described in this chapter was the introduction in 1976 of a comprehensive planning system for English health and personal social services. One of the purposes of the system was to secure higher priority for services that directly benefit the elderly.

The planning system is only one element of a larger innovation that involved establishing structures for health-service management, decision-making processes, and principles for resource allocation. Because these structures, processes, and principles are interrelated, they are explained briefly in paragraphs 1–20. Paragraphs 21–44 describe in more detail the attempt to give priority to services for the elderly and the outcome of that attempt. Paragraph 45 is a brief note on the reward system established.

A. GENERAL

The National Health Service (NHS)

1. Britain has had a National Health Service since 1948. Its objective is to provide comprehensive health care, largely free of charge. Nearly all hospitals and clinics are owned by the state and are financed from general taxation. Hospital doctors are salaried, although many senior doc-

tors opt for a form of contract that allows them to spend part of their time on private practice. The great majority of general practitioners "contract" to give services to NHS patients and draw most of their incomes from the state. Doctors and other health professionals continuously complain about underfunding; expenditure on health care in Britain has indeed grown more slowly than in many other countries. Other critics of the NHS point to continuing regional inequalities or assert that too large a share of resources has been given to high-technology medicine at the expense of preventive medicine, primary care, and supportive services for the elderly, the mentally ill, and the handicapped. For the latter groups, there is a difficult boundary line between the responsibilities of the NHS and those of local authorities who provide domestic assistance, community homes, and social-work services.

Integration

2. The 1948 administrative structure of the NHS was fragmented, for example, separate, ad hoc agencies were set up to administer groups of teaching and nonteaching hospitals. They were given no responsibility for health services in the community and often had to operate in ill-defined or overlapping catchment areas. Central control was very weak. Gradually, however, the need for coordination between hospital and other services (especially services for the elderly and the mentally ill) was realized. There was also concern about the mounting cost of high-technology hospital medicine and the underdevelopment of services for chronic and degenerative patients. Professional, political, and administrative interests joined forces to achieve a more integrated system of administration, which was implemented in 1974, on the same date that a general reorganization of local government was instituted.

3. One of the objectives of the NHS reorganization was to give the central department more opportunity to plan and influence the general direction of developments, particularly in a manner that would favor the interests of vulnerable ("cinderella") patient groups. Another objective was to establish area-health authorities with comprehensive responsibility to plan and provide services to meet the needs of a defined geographical population. In general, these populations were coterminous with those eligible for personal social services from the relevant tier of local government. These services had been combined into integrated social-service departments (covering the social needs of children, the mentally ill, the aged, the handicapped, et al.) some years earlier. Health and local-government authorities were required by statute to collaborate and set up joint committees.[1,2,3]

Structure

4. The Department of Health and Social Security (DHSS) oversees both health and social-service authorities. Although the secretary of state is considered responsible for the NHS, he is responsible only for the general direction and adequacy of local-authority services. He appoints members of fourteen regional-health authorities (RHAs) and the chairmen of ninety area-health authorities (AHAs). Other members of area authorities are appointed by the RHAs. Various professional and other interests have to be accommodated in the membership, and at least one-third of both bodies are nominated by local-government authorities. The chairmen are paid part-time salaries; other members are not paid.

5. Each authority appoints its own staff. RHAs (which have no local-government counterpart) are responsible for planning services for populations of about three million and for supervising the constituent planning services within their areas, for operating them on a day-to-day basis, and for collaborating with local authorities. (The use of the word *planning* to explain the functions of all three levels will be explained later.)

6. Within each area decision processes are structured around management teams and consultative machinery. (In fact, most areas are subdivided into districts, but we shall take the simpler case.) Immediately below the area-health authority is an area-management team, consisting of four permanent officers (the area-medical officer, the nursing officer, the administrator, and the treasurer) who are appointed by the authority and two doctors (one hospital specialist and one general practitioner) who are elected by their peers. All members have to agree on decisions. The composition of these teams was decided nationally after negotiations with the health professions. The intentions were:

a. that the main health professions should be represented in management;

b. that there should be an equal voice for hospital and nonhospital medicine;

c. that the community-health interest should be represented by the area-medical officer.

7. In addition to the management team, there are four kinds of bodies with which an area-health authority has to consult about major proposals:

a. separate professional advisory committees, whose memberships are balanced to reflect hospital and community interests, for medical, dental, nursing, optical, and pharmacological staffs;

b. consultative committees, representing organized staff groups (mainly ambulance personnel, ancillary workers, and clerical staff);
c. community-health councils, which consist of lay people (some from local authorities and some from voluntary organizations concerned with health), whose tasks involve representing the interests of the community served by the health authority;
d. the statutory joint consultative committee with local authorities.

8. For some services there are planning teams that either work with the area-management team or, on joint planning questions, with the joint AHA/local authority consultative committee. The structure is shown in Figure 12.1

Finance

9. In January or February of each year, the government publishes a white paper on public expenditure. This report covers public spending as a whole, projected for the coming financial year and usually for four ad-

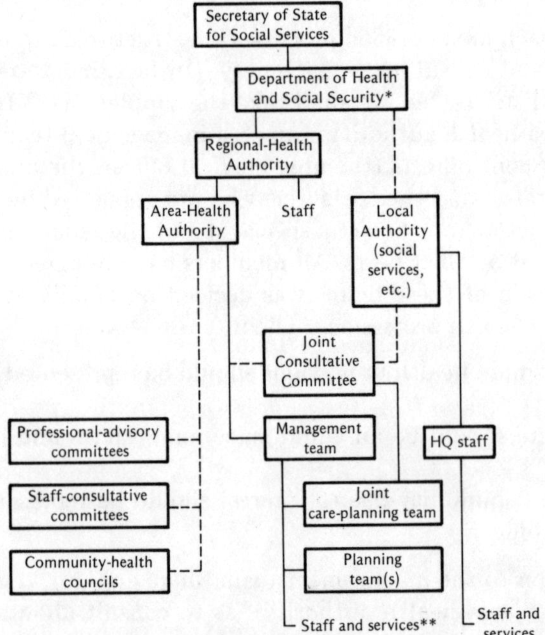

*DHSS is also responsible, through separate regional and local offices, for administering cash social-security benefits.
**Family-practitioner services are not administered by the management teams but by a semiautonomous committee on which the practitioners are strongly represented.

Figure 12.1

ditional years, for fifteen "Programmes." Although matters seldom turn out as projected in the white paper, the report is intended to serve three main purposes:

a. It signals government intentions for public spending as a whole and supplies the expenditure side of the budget statement issued in the spring;
b. By projecting future needs from past trends (technically very difficult in inflationary conditions), it shows how priorities are to be shifted for individual programs such as defense, roads and transport, housing, social security, and so on.
c. It shows how programs are made up and sets forth reasons for projected increases and decreases (e.g., the effect of changes in population on education programs, or the effect of policy changes).

10. The production of the white paper is partly a technical exercise. But its final shape is highly political, for the main programs match the responsibilities of powerful cabinet ministers and determine how much they and their departments will have to spend in the coming year. For example, the white paper of January 1978 allowed for only a 2.1 percent growth (in real terms) of the health and personal-services (HPSS) program per annum from 1976–1977 to 1981–1982.[4] This increase allows very little room for new policies or even for expanding the existing level of services to accommodate, for example, the growing numbers over the age of 75, who are heavy users of these services. Social and economic priorities come together in the white paper. It is therefore an exercise, however crude, in macroplanning among sectors.

11. The health and personal social-services (HPSS) program amounts to about 15 percent of public expenditure on goods and services and almost 7 percent of national income. Ignoring the complicating details, the program falls into two parts: (a) the NHS (b) personal social services.

12. The NHS part of the program is spent by the government itself. Most of it is earmarked for hospital and community-health services and is divided among regional-health authorities, who in turn allocate most of their shares among area-health authorities. In recent years, a formula has been worked out for allocating money strictly on the basis of the population served by each authority, with extra points given for high mortality and for unusual age compositions. But because of past inequalities, such as the overprovision of expensive hospital beds in London, these allocations are only "targets" that cannot be implemented. Regional-health authorities that are spending more than their "target" allocations are given very little more than the previous year's allocations. The increase in the national budget is used mainly to help the poorer regions. At a time when overall growth is very small, this method

of allocation has caused great bitterness and argument and has generated hostility to planning as well.

13. The personal social-services part of HPSS is what the government would like local authorities to spend on those services. Although it is not a government grant, it is included, along with similar estimates for education, housing, and other services provided by local authorities, in an estimate of total local-government expenditures that the government will "recognize" for grant aid. The government then decides what proportion of that total will be grant aided (usually about 60 percent). The grant is paid in block to individual local authorities on a different (and very complex) formula based on indices of need. It is changed slightly every year for political reasons (for example, if the government wishes to give more help to London, other large cities, and localities). The important point is that the planned expenditure on personal social services is "lost" in the global allocation. The government cannot make individual local authorities spend their grants in ways that would make the public-expenditure sums come out right. (In fact, spending on personal social services often exceeds the sum that the government intended.)

14. Finally, the government has even less control over how local authorities spend their money *within* the personal social services (i. e., among different patient groups). The only controls have been directed toward buildings, and the general policy is to relax specific controls that would prevent a local authority from building children's homes when the government wished to give priority to old people's homes.

15. There is a separation between capital expenditure and running costs. Large building schemes are controlled, and money is earmarked for certain kinds of development. For example, regional-health authorities are expected to spend stated percentages of their capital-development money on centers for primary medical care. Some money can be used only to fund local-authority services that relieve the burden on hospitals. But most of the allocation is free from constraint. Large global sums are therefore spent at the discretion of individual health authorities, who are, of course, constrained by decisions of the past—existing hospital patterns, commitments to staff, and so forth.

Planning

16. One of the purposes of the 1974 reorganization was to increase the central direction of strategic policy, while leaving as much discretion as possible to regional and area-health authorities. Borrowing from corporate planning in large industry, the circle was to be squared by means of a "planning cycle" in which lower-tier authorities would prepare detailed plans within strategic guidelines issued by higher-tier authorities. If the

plans were consistent with the guidelines, they would be approved, and the authorities would then be accountable for implementing them. But the guidelines would themselves be kept under review in light of actual experience.

17. Because of political changes and administrative delays, the first set of guidelines was not issued by DHSS until March 1976.[5] They state the government's policies for different aspects of health care (for example, the policy of caring for the mentally handicapped in the community instead of in hospitals, and the policy of using hospital facilities more efficiently in order to reduce waiting lists for surgery). None of these policies was new. But the guidelines brought them together for the first time and suggested priorities. Specifically, they contained analyses of the projected figures in the HPSS public-expenditure program and explanations of how spending for some services would have to rise and spending for others would have to fall in order to progress toward priority objectives within the total sum of resources likely to be available. Regional-health authorities were asked to consider these suggestions and to propose ways of implementing them within their regions. But the major task of adapting the strategies to local circumstances was to rest with the area-health authorities and their management and planning teams. The AHAs would have to take into account guidelines from the RHA as well as those from DHSS. Instructions from an AHA to its officers could include further policy guidance (although in practice any policies adopted by the lay, part-time authority members would probably have been initiated by the management team).

18. All this concerns *strategic* planning, that is, the progressive application of general principles to local circumstances, at the three levels, DHSS, RHA, and AHA. Translating strategies into staff and services ("operational planning") is separate from and logically subordinate to "strategic planning."

19. Planning instructions prescribed the way in which area-strategic plans were to be prepared. The management teams were expected to prepare draft plans in light of (a) the policy guidelines that had been issued to them (b) their knowledge of local situations. The draft plan was supposed to include, for example, statistics showing special local needs and comparisons of local services with averages and "norms" for the region and for the country as a whole; this exercise would enable others to ascertain how the proposals in the plans would help overcome known deficiencies. All the bodies mentioned in paragraph 7 would have to be consulted about the draft plan. Their comments had to be taken into account or else had to be reported to the authority when it considered the draft. The final area-strategic plan would be proposed after considering all these comments and then forwarded to the regional authority.

20. After a similar process of consultation with professional advisory committees at the regional level, the RHA was to approve or disapprove the area plans. The parts that were approved (because they were consistent with the guidelines) were combined into a regional plan and forwarded for approval by DHSS. This was done for the first time early in 1977. The first progress report shows that the plan was not complete. Moreover, local plans showed marked inconsistencies with national objectives.[6] Although the original intention had been to conduct the strategic-planning exercise only every third year, it was agreed that because the plans were so incomplete, a further attempt would be made in 1978–1979. In the meantime, of course, changes in staff and services continued on a year-to-year basis, even if they were inconsistent with the overall strategy.

B. SERVICES FOR THE ELDERLY

The Problem

21. The improvement of services for the elderly was frequently mentioned as an objective of the structural and procedural reforms mentioned in the preceding section. Since the 1950s, it has been pointed out that the number of old people in the population is increasing and that additional resources will have to be found to meet their needs.[7] Demographic figures are readily available and are used every year by the secretary of state in his annual battle with other ministers to secure an increase in the HPSS program. (See paragraph 10.) However, the parliamentary committee that reviews government expenditure pointed out in 1972 that there was no evidence that the resources approved by Parliament for this purpose were actually being used to benefit the elderly rather than health services in general.[8]

22. Second, it was believed that health services for the elderly were being neglected in order to finance high-technology medicine. Surveys and research studies suggested that existing services were meeting only a small part of the total need.[9,10] Moreover, a series of scandals, commencing with a private letter to *The Times* in 1965, attracted public interest in the conditions under which elderly patients were being treated in hospitals catering to long stays.[11] These disclosures activated a number of pressure groups and led directly to the creation of an inspection service to promote higher standards[12] (in contradiction to the general philosophy that the local administration of health care could safely be left to the local-agent authorities and their professional staffs).

23. Third, the needs of the elderly played a prominent part in the argu-

ments about administrative unification: It was believed that their needs transcended hospital and community boundaries and that effective provision required better coordination of services under unified authorities. (The evidence for this conclusion is very meager, and in any case the logic has not been pursued because the medical, social, housing, and financial needs of the elderly continue to be met by different agencies operating under different criteria.)

The Political Market

24. There is no doctrinal dispute between the main political parties about the needs of the elderly. Conservative and Labour ministers have made almost identical speeches about their plight and the need for rectification. In political terms, the elderly are supported by the general climate of opinion. The mass media give good coverage to the problems of the elderly and in particular to deficiencies in state services. Several pressure groups campaign vigorously on their behalf. The Trade Union Congress passes annual resolutions in favor of higher pensions and better services (somewhat unrealistically, for the cost has to be met from the living standards of current wage earners; but the British trade-union movement has tended to look to the state rather than to employers for retirement provisions).

25. This concern, however, is not matched within professional structures. In medicine, geriatrics is recognized as a specialty. But it fails to attract enough doctors, in spite of good career prospects and the limited number of posts in more glamorous branches of medicine. Geriatrics has low status and tends to be staffed by immigrant doctors. Nurses and paramedical workers prefer to work with acutely ill patients who have chances of recovery rather than with the intractable conditions of old age. Even social workers are more attracted by preventive work with children than by ameliorative work with the elderly and the handicapped.

National Planning

26. Within DHSS the responsibility for developing policies for the elderly belongs to a special team within the service development group. It includes a doctor, a nurse, a social worker, and an administrator. Its function is to develop policies for the elderly within the health and personal social services. The team briefs ministers for parliamentary debates and speeches. It deals with pressure groups. It is represented at important conferences on the elderly. It is the "customer" for a large program of research on the elderly and their service needs, a program

that operates through an academic "research liaison group." It is in contact with other departments about formulating a statement of government policies toward the elderly, including housing, employment, and income requirements, which will be published (in 1978) to stimulate discussion and innovation. (Each health authority in England will be invited to comment on the document, as is the custom, when it is published, and reactions will be taken into account in the final statement of policy.) But perhaps the most important function of the service development team is to prepare those parts of the national planning guidelines that relate to the elderly.

27. We are not concerned here with the content of those plans but with the priority accorded to them within the total health and personal social-service framework. Priority is established in the context of resources. A central-planning group compares the cost of proposals to develop services for the elderly with the cost of other proposals that have to be met from the HPSS program. Within the projected growth of that program, decisions are made about which services should be encouraged to develop at a faster or a slower rate and which, if any, should be cut back. For example, the 1976 guidelines assumed an overall growth rate of about two percent per annum over a four-year period in the sum available for running costs of the HPSS program. Within that total, growth rates for particular services were calculated as follows (it being assumed that growth at the recommended rate would enable specific policies for each group to be achieved):

Primary care services	+ 3.8 percent
Services for the elderly (and younger handicapped)	+ 3.2 percent
Services for the mentally handicapped	+ 2.8 percent
Services for children and families	+ 2.2 percent
Services for the mentally ill	+ 1.8 percent
Acute and general-hospital services	+ 1.2 percent
Hospital-maternity services	– 1.8 percent

28. These figures were not imposed on the health authorities. It was recognized that circumstances and existing levels of provision would vary from place to place. (In 1975–1976, for example, regional expenditure on health services for the elderly varied from £64 to £41 per person aged 65 and over.) But the authorities were asked to include in their plans specific policies that, when aggregated, would be consistent with these figures.

29. The following situation confronted the health authorities:

a. The budget from which they had to meet the costs of existing services as well as new ones was fixed on a basis that allowed little or no overall growth in the rich London regions and only slow growth in the poorer regions. (See paragraph 12.)

b. If their services for priority groups, including the elderly, were deficient (as measured against such "norms" as the ratio of geriatric hospital beds per thousand of elderly patients), they were expected to improve them at a faster rate than the general level of development.

c. They were expected to achieve this improvement by expanding acute hospital services at a slower rate than the general level of development (at a much slower rate than in the past) and by *reducing* expenditure for maternity services, which had continued to increase in spite of a continuing decline in the number of births since 1964. (Between 1970 and 1973 the birthrate fell by 15 percent, but expenditure for hospital maternity cases rose by nearly the same amount.) The success of the plan for the elderly would depend on the determination of the health authorities to reverse the expansionist tendencies of other services.

The Local Political Market

30. Regional health authorities are not important for this discussion, although planning is an important part of their raison d'être. RHAs are a distance from the battlefront. In the *downward* part of the planning process, most of them played their expected roles by reviewing the quality of services in the region against the DHSS guidelines and by advising the area-health authorities on their applicability to local conditions. RHAs have statistical and other planning capacities to carry out such exercises and are in regular, close contact both with their constituent AHAs and with DHSS. The authorities, however, defend their regions and resources against the DHSS. Their structures of professional advisory committees and lay members open them to pressure from dissatisfied AHAs and staff. Their ability to respond to such pressures in a planning rather than in a political way is more doubtful in the *upward* than in the downward parts of the process. In the downward parts of the process, they are dealing with generalizations and technological rationalizations. In the upward parts, they have to listen to angry people who are not getting what they want.

31. It was at the area level that planning had to take root if it was to be effective. The major objective of the planning system was to secure commitments from area-health authorities to strategies that were consistent with national-planning strategies in the circumstances of particular areas. The *structure* described in paragraphs 6–8 was intended to create an environment in which the AHAs would receive balanced advice. For

example, one would suppose that policies designed to develop services for the elderly, rather than high-technology medicine, would be supported by:

a. the joint-consultative committee and its joint care-planning team on which health-authority members and their staffs discuss common problems with the local authority that provides the elderly with social services;
b. the area medical officer in his capacity as "community physician" and expert in demographic and social medicine;
c. general practitioners and other community-health professionals who balance the hospital-based professionals on every management team, on the professional-advisory committee, and, indeed, on the authority itself;
d. representatives on community-health councils of organizations concerned with the elderly.

32. Moreover, the planning process, which stresses the need for consultation with all these groups as well as with staff representatives, was intended to *involve* each of these putative spokesmen and to provide them with *information* (norms, guidelines, existing levels of provision) that they could deploy in the political debate. Consultation was based on the assumption that (a) the actual process would be comprehensive, (b) people would play the parts expected of them, and (c) they would be able to handle the analytic (especially the statistical) material that constitutes the basis for strategic planning.

33. In practice, none of these assumptions was justified.[13] In most areas, there was neither time nor the analytic resources necessary to prepare the analytic material or to go through the full consultative process prescribed in the DHSS planning manual in 1976–1977. One authority that attempted to complete the process produced a thick, heavily annotated document containing draft plans, commentary by various bodies, and comments on the commentary by the officers who had prepared the draft. AHA members were unable to digest so much material. Some resolved the overload problem by yielding to the strongest political forces. Others accepted the technological (and political) judgments of their principal officers.

34. Nor did the political balance of forces work out as expected:

a. Local-authority participants in the planning process were in a weak position because there were more deficiencies on the social-services side than in health-authority provisions for the elderly.
b. Area medical officers are not necessarily trained in demographic and social medicine. Moreover, other aspects of their roles, includ-

ing their responsibilities for medical staffing and for the efficient use of hospital resources, compel them to maintain good relations with powerful specialists in high-technology medicine.

c. In practice, the authority of community-health professionals is weak compared to that of hospital-based professionals. Again, general practitioners and community nurses have professional incentives (working relationships, career prospects) for not opposing developments in high-technology medicine. In any case, their interests in community services do not necessarily coincide with concern for the elderly and other priority groups.

d. Finally, the role of community-health councils was equally unpredictable. At least one council played a significant part. In an area that was very short of geriatric hospital beds, a teaching hospital was built. The doctors and management teams wanted to allocate all the beds to high-technology medicine. But the community-health council, skillfully using information provided by the regional planners, fought a successful battle to have some beds allocated to geriatrics. Other community-health councils aligned themselves with high-technology medicine. Council members were often concerned about deficiencies in acute hospital services; they criticized economy campaigns directed at these services and provided a focal point for resistance to the closure of small maternity hospitals that were underused and could be closed in order to release resources to develop priority services.

35. The political-market assumption neglected two important factors. One was the salience of high-technology specialists in the whole health-care system. Many analysts have shown that investment in high-technology medicine produces diminishing returns.[14] But the prestige of cardiac surgeons and gastroenterologists, for example, is very high. If one of them claims that a new piece of equipment or the appointment of additional diagnostic staff will save individual lives, few of his fellow professionals, let alone lay authority members, have enough technical knowledge to argue against him. Many will be emotionally disposed to accept his arguments. The second neglected factor was the power and motivation of staff groups. It is well-known that any change creates a threat to established interests, which will therefore oppose it. Any slow-down of high-technology medicine is a threat to the career prospects of those groups that are linked with it. Any increase in efficiency suggests more effort or at least the adoption of different methods by some groups of staff. Most seriously, any proposal to close an inefficient hospital creates a threat to those who work in it, from nurses to porters and domestic workers. In Britain today, where trade unions have immense power (and,

given the unemployment situation, every incentive to use it to protect their jobs), it is the unskilled, ancillary workers who mobilize resources against the closure of surplus maternity units.

36. The third assumption was that analytic information would be deployed to counteract the validity of the argument paragraphs. All the evidence is that this assumption was unrealistic. In the first place, few people are intellectually equipped to deal with statistics and abstractions: The representative of a voluntary organization on a community-health council is more interested in anecdotal information about transport facilities, hygiene, or discharge procedures than about demographic trends. Second, the analytic material was often not available. Finally, those who received it were often unaware of its significance.

37. In general, nobody is opposed to the development of services for the elderly. It is therefore easy for members of area-health authorities and other bodies to pass resolutions affirming their intention of improving services (e. g., chiropody) when circumstances and resources permit. It is quite another thing to accept the fact that within a limited budget, the development of these services affects alternative objectives. The same authorities that passed pious resolutions in support of services for the elderly committed themselves to other developments that in effect made it impossible to achieve their objectives for the elderly.

38. In such an arena, the role of information was subordinated to political considerations. Even when information was available, it was either neglected or disputed when it did not fit the interests of a campaigning group. For example, one management team tried to demonstrate that a small maternity hospital was not needed. They produced figures showing that the hospital had very few patients, other maternity hospitals could meet this level of demand, and a certain sum of money could be saved by the closure of the hospital. Opponents claimed that the estimates of future birthrates were too low; they alleged that the savings had been exaggerated; they ignored the evidence about low occupancy and changed the argument by focusing on amenity and accessibility.

39. Part of the problem was that the local people were much more interested in operational problems than in strategic planning. There was no way of securing their commitment to a strategy in advance of working out its detailed consequences. Strategic policies were either accepted without question because they were considered too general to have any real meaning or they were ignored in the battle to protect or advance specific developments.

The Local Plans

40. Local plans, therefore, often included some vague statements, agreeing in principle with the national objectives. But a statement of

support was usually followed by a list of high-technology services that the local people had always wanted. Among the arguments advanced against giving immediate priority to the elderly were the following:

a. We do not accept the priority. First consideration should be given to the needs of the working population who suffer from acute illness.
b. We need more money. We would like to do more for the elderly but not at the expense of high-technology services.
c. Give us time. We can save money by rationalizing high-technology services. But this strategy needs investment, and so, for the next few years, we shall be spending *more* on high technology.
d. The planning assumptions are incorrect. The elderly will benefit more from the general development of services than from giving priority to services that are specific to them (e. g., hospital geriatrics).
e. The figures are incorrect. Technical mistakes in categorizing expenditure give misleading impressions. The demographic projections are wrong (e. g., it is unwise to plan for a low birthrate).
f. Quality is more important than quantity.

Completing the Cycle

41. Regional-health authorities had to compare area plans with broad strategies and to combine them into a regional plan. This procedure proved almost impossible. Regions could not do the work assigned to the AHAs, even though they had better analytic resources. Nor could they impose their own plans on the AHAs. All they could do was try to make the plans look rational, cutting out any proposal that could not be met within the total resource expectations. What finally reached the central department (DHSS) from the regions was a set of proposals, mostly for capital development, accompanied by statements about good intentions and long lists of reasons why it was impossible to implement the national strategy in the short term.

42. In light of this development, DHSS produced a further discussion document in September 1977.[15] Some imperfections in the original guidelines were admitted. But it was claimed that some parts of the previous document had been misunderstood. The secretary of state reaffirmed his policy about priorities. He acknowledged the fact that health authorities were facing many difficulties and that progress would be slower than had been hoped. At about that time, the HPSS program again came under review by the parliamentary committee on expenditure. The committee looked at the limited success of the planning initiative and commented that only time would tell whether the outcome would be any different from what the health authorities, left to themselves, would have done.[16]

43. Subsequently, statistics for 1976–1977 (the year in which the guidelines were considered) showed that:

a. expenditure for hospital services increased, whereas expenditure for community services (including chiropody) decreased;
b. the number of hospital geriatric cases increased, whereas expenditure per case decreased;
c. the number of births fell again, but the cost per hospital delivery increased and total expenditures for maternity services appear not to have fallen.[17]

Summary

44. Analyses of demographic trends and service standards led to a national policy of according priority to certain services for the elderly. Area-health authorities were asked to prepare local plans for putting this strategy into effect. But the health authorities were faced with different problems and found reasons or excuses for adopting different policies. Short of actually telling the area authorities what to do, the DHSS could only accept the situation and resort to further persuasion. The success of the first attempt at rational planning to meet the needs of the elderly within the National Health Service was therefore very limited. (Similar difficulty was experienced in securing priority for the elderly within local-authority budgets.)

C. NOTE ON THE REWARD SYSTEM

45. The reward system has not played any part in this innovation, although it is relevant to attracting medical and other resources to caring for the elderly. Nurses who work in geriatric, chronic, and hospitals catering to long stays have received pay supplements since 1968. General practitioners are paid a mixture of allowances, capitation fees, fees per item of service, and reimbursement of expenses. Since 1966, a higher capitation fee has been paid for patients over 65; but this increase was intended as compensation for extra work rather than as an inducement. Hospital doctors receive the same salary, regardless of specialty. Geriatricians, however, are less able than doctors in the acute specialties to augment their incomes with private practices, and they are less likely to receive "distinction awards" (which are conferred by a panel sitting in secret and, at the highest level of award, can double a consultant's salary). In 1974, the government proposed that doctors working in shortage specialties, including geriatrics, and in unpopular areas should receive

additional reward; but negotiations with the profession broke down, and the proposal was abandoned after doctors had taken industrial action in protest against some aspects of the package. The fact remains that too many doctors want to become surgeons and cardiologists, and too few want to become geriatricians. Some attempt is being made to change this imbalance by restricting the number of training posts in the popular specialties. Medical graduates are also being made aware of the greater opportunities for promotion in specialties such as geriatrics.

REFERENCES

1. *National Health Service Reorganisation: England.* (Cmnd. 5055). London: HMSO, 1972.
2. National Health Service Reorganisation Act, 1973.
3. National Health Service Act, 1977.
4. *The Government's Expenditure Plans, 1978–1979 to 1981–1982.* (Cmnd. 7049). London: HMSO, 1978.
5. Department of Health and Social Security. *Priorities for Health and Personal Social Services in England.* London: HMSO, 1976.
6. Department of Health and Social Security. *The Way Forward.* London: HMSO, 1977.
7. Report of the Committee on the Economic and Financial Problems of the Provision for Old Age. (Cmd. 9333). London: HMSO, 1954.
8. Eighth Report of the Expenditure Committee for 1971–1972. "The Relationship of Expenditure to Needs," HC 575, 1971–1972.
9. Office of Population Censuses and Surveys. *The General Household Survey: Introductory Report.* London: HMSO, 1973 (and subsequent).
10. Hunt, Audrey. *The Elderly at Home.* London: HMSO, 1978.
11. Robb, Barbara. ed. *Sans Everything: A Case to Answer.* Nelson, 1967.
12. Crossman, Richard. *Diaries of a Cabinet Minister,* vol. III, 1968–1970. London: Hamish Hamilton and Jonathan Cape, 1977. (See index under Hospitals and Hospital advisory service.)
13. This material is based on research in the field and on *The Way Forward, op. cit.*
14. Cochrane, A. L. *Effectiveness and Efficiency: Random Reflections on Health Services.* Nuffield Provincial Hospitals Trust, 1972.
15. *The Way Forward, op. cit.*
16. Ninth Report of the Expenditure Committee for 1976–1977. "Spending on the Health and Personal Social Services," HC 466, 1976–1977.
17. Department of Health and Social Services. Circular HC(78)12. "DHSS Planning Guidelines for 1978–1979." March 1978.

Chapter 13

Innovative Policy for Central-Local Government Cooperation in the Finnish Health System

A. S. Härö

A. INTRODUCTION

Health and medical care are service sectors in which innovations are more the rule than the exception. This observation pertains to drugs, diagnostic methods, and forms of treatment. On the other hand, innovative actions that aim at developing the service system are much less common. A 1973 World Health Assembly proclaimed that there is much justified dissatisfaction about the organization of service systems.[1] Especially now, when developing countries confront the dilemma of allocating very limited resources to meet very great needs for services, experience acquired in devising innovative solutions to the organization of primary care is invaluable.

This chapter focuses attention on a recent national-level innovation. In 1972 the concept of a primary health center was introduced in Finland through special legislation designed to reshape the primary health services. In a very short time, the whole nation was served by such centers. This analysis, written in 1978, is directed toward evaluating the progress of "introducing innovations." The focus of interest centers on how the innovative reshaping was initiated, directed, and so on. Less attention is given to such material achievements as the volume of services performed and other comparable aspects.

Progress evaluation was defined in the working document of the World Health Assembly (31st, 1978) in the following way:[2]

> . . . is concerned with the comparison of the actual with the scheduled programme delivery, the identification of reasons for achievements or shortcomings, and indications for remedies for any shortcomings. The purpose of a progress review is to facilitate the monitoring and operational control of ongoing activities. In terms of systems analysis it is a review of the use of "inputs."

B. THE PLAN OF THIS CHAPTER

Three objectives guided the preparation of this chapter. Primary health care is an acute problem in most developing countries. Therefore, to describe innovative approaches in this field is a valid objective. The introduction of program budgeting in a country that has very strong traditions of decentralized decision making is another innovation that deserves attention. But perhaps the third objective is most important: to evaluate how these innovations were introduced. This objective was pursued with the aid of the framework used in an international study conducted by the OECD: "Policies for Innovation in the Service Sector".[3] The study focused attention on situations in which changes were systematically introduced. Primary health services in Finland constituted one of the case studies.[4] The framework relates to the following points:

1. problem perception and formulation
2. the environment
3. the initiating unit
4. the innovation
5. techniques of change
6. adopters and users
7. the impact of the innovation

Some knowledge of Finnish society, especially the organization of health services, should illuminate this case study. The first section of this chapter is intended to provide that knowledge.

C. SOME ORGANIZATIONAL ASPECTS OF THE FINNISH HEALTH-CARE SYSTEM

In Finland, as in other Scandinavian countries, health services and medical care are considered obligations of society and the natural right of citizen. This right is not limited to the poor but devolves on the whole population. This attitude is widespread, and so it is not surprising that health is not at all mentioned in the Finnish constitution. The health-service system has been built on a substructure of local authorities. These "communes" have elected (by means of proportional representation) councils and exercise marked autonomy in various fields, including finance. They also have the right to levy income tax. If some exceptions are ignored, rural and urban communities have the same rights and responsibilities. In principle, these communes are the basic units of the system. The councils are responsible for organizing services. Small local units form joint bodies to provide services. Decentralized administration based on small, autonomic local authority seems to satisfy the democratic expectations of Finnish society, and the policy of giving organizational responsibility to small local units was devised to achieve an equitable distribution of basic services.

Another objective was "direct consumer control" to be achieved through the (proportionally) elected council. Basic services are mainly paid for by tax revenue, but there is also an obligatory national health insurance that covers the use of private physicians, transportation, and so on. In general, the private sector is relatively small in Finland. Executive powers and responsibility for care are, to a great extent, decentralized, but supervision and direction are markedly centralized. The central government is influential in three major ways. It licenses physicians and other key personnel as well as institutions such as hospitals. Another means of influence is related to the right to know. In Finland this right covers the expenditure of tax money for any purpose whatsoever. Knowledge is a strong power especially when it is linked with financial arrangements, which constitute the third method of influence. In Finland costs are divided between local and central authorities. The central government usually subsidizes communes by paying 50 percent of the total (accepted) expenditure. The central government can invoke economic sanctions, for instance, by refusing to pay its part of the expenditure. In such cases the local authority is not prevented from acting but must take full responsibility for economic consequences.

If applied together, these measures provide considerable scope for regulatory actions. But there is one obvious restriction: The central government cannot dictate what local authorities should do. The central government can issue directives only if parliament enacts a special law. But passing such legislation is difficult because of the strict minority clauses in the basic laws of the country. Parliament considers very carefully the opinions of local authorities. Many members of parliament are active politicians at the local authority level.

D. INTRODUCING INNOVATIONS

Problem Perception and Formulation

Before planned organizational change can be initiated, problems must be perceived. In Finland no series of actions to make the nation aware of the shortcomings of primary care was noticeable, but increasingly dramatic titles of critiques signaled the growth of this perception:

"The Population of Finland—The Sickest in Europe"
"The Healthiest Children—The Unhealthiest Men" [5]

WHO data on life expectancy, international comparisons based on the standard mortality rate (SMR), and infant mortality rates were cited as evidence. These kinds of articles, both in medical periodicals as well as in newspapers, led to the contention that one of the main reasons for the shortcomings was to be found in the primary services. Considerable inequity characterized primary care, and problems were accentuated in less developed areas of the country.

One can say that there existed considerable "outside pressure" for change. "Internal" pressure was generated by the growth of budgeted hospital expenditure. A frequent critique was based on the contention that the volume of hospital services was too large. The basic problem was perceived to be the lack of balance between primary, nonhospital health care and secondary, hospital-based services. Another aspect of the same problem derived from the fact that too many service subsystems at the local level were based on special laws or ad hoc arrangements that made functioning ineffective and coordinating actions difficult. A related problem was the lack of a suitable mechanism that could facilitate close cooperation on the part of local and central government officials. The planning horizon—one budgetary year—was too short for implementing purposeful manpower policy and accumulating greater investments. Awareness of the problem had grown to such an extent by 1965 that a state committee was appointed to plan the reorganization of primary care. Its report, published in 1967, increased awareness of the urgency of the problems by formulating it more precisely and by proposing some possible solutions.

Corrective action was to be taken to achieve the following objectives:

to construct an organizational structure for introducing required innovations (organizational output);
to build a mechanism that would facilitate national control over critical issues (control output);
to increase the volume of services (volume output);

to revise objectives for existing services (subject-matter output);
to achieve areal and social equity (distributional output).

In addition, numerous minor or secondary outputs often served to make progress possible. Examples are the innovation of devising a salary system for physicians, standardizing the educational requirements for nurses, nurse-midwives, and numerous other categories of personnel. Another output was the relatively rapid abolition of all direct charges for primary care.

The Environment: Developmental Strategies

Problems are perceived within an environmental context, and in many cases changes are formulated to conform to specific environments. But many other prerequisites exist. There must be a reasonably well-functioning political decision-making system, money, manpower, and mental resources that can be mobilized. In Finland the environment was suitable for innovative actions. There was space for "disjointed incrementalism",[6] but basic problems could not be solved without restructuring the organization. Accordingly, much attention was devoted to organizational problems.

Although the list of problems is not exhaustive, it reflects the picture perceived by responsible authorities and politicians. The outputs labeled *control, volume, subject-matter,* and *distributional* derive from the *organizational* output. The key issue was how to strengthen the role of the central authorities in a country that has a political and an administrative tradition of decentralization.

In principle, three strategies were examined:

to rely on local incremental decisions without resorting to major regulatory measures;
to strengthen the powers of the central government;
to innovate the rules governing the interplay between the central and local governments.

The first alternative would neither promote nor improve areal inequities. Small local authorities cannot assume major responsibility for national problems such as manpower shortages, curative services, and so on.

The second alternative could be evaluated on the basis of experience. Until World War II, the central government tried to solve comparable problems by making direct investments in selected projects in less developed areas, in isolated islands, and so on. This approach solved some of the most urgent difficulties, but the managerial rigidity of the central government inhibited the development of comprehensive services in which local and central interests could be linked. Relying on the central government would reverse the traditional policy of decentralizing decision making in the social-service sector.

The third alternative—the interplay strategy—was, in principle, the most promising, but some requirement would have to be devised to ensure central government guidance without generating negative side effects. A modified version of PPBS (planning-programming-budgeting system) was adopted,[7] and special legislation was enacted. The goal was an organizational configuration that would facilitate coordinated planning at the national and local levels.

The Initiating Unit

Health services constitute "risk services" provided to individuals to cope with conditions over which they have little control. The provision rests on some form of consensus that can be translated into actions.

The introduction of an innovation normally follows a chain of events. Some are conceptual and relate to the perception of problems. The development of a concrete plan of action sometimes indicates who has initiated the process. At the national level, innovations that require legislation are usually initiated by units that are responsible for initiation and implementation.

It is hardly possible in Finland to initiate the planning of a major reorganization from the bottom up; the main initiative must come from the top level. The power to effect reorganization resides in the cabinet, which is the only alternative to a formal initiator. Primary health care was cited as one of the political goals of the cabinet for the first time in 1968. The proposal of the committee (1967) was taken as the starting point, and a planning commission was appointed. It was composed of high-level administrators and included the political secretary of the minister of health. It cooperated closely with other ministers in the cabinet and produced a revised proposal for legislation. Each subsequent cabinet has proclaimed that primary care will continue to be developed.

Because of the important roles played by the national and local governments in providing and financing health care, it is hardly reasonable to expect that any informal pressure group, such as physicians, could play a central role in the initiating process. No insurance system exists that could gain from rearranging services.

The problems were perceived directly at the local authority level, but local authorities do not have enough political and other tangible resources to initiate actions, and, in addition, a consensus is very difficult to achieve at that level. There are urban and rural authorities, some located in big university centers and others located in "developing" areas. Members of various local councils belong to different political parties, and political divisions, among other reasons, make very difficult the formulation of local-authority initiatives.

E. THE INNOVATIONS

Innovative Aspects of Legislation

Decisive for successful planning in the social field is a framework that would make the activity possible and acceptable to all parties concerned. In Finnish society, because of the autonomy of local authorities, only legislation approved by parliament can serve as such a framework. As previously mentioned, a specific law concerning primary health (no. 66/72) was passed at the beginning of 1972. The time—about four months—reserved for its introduction was very short. The brevity of the time span involved seemed to have provoked a "crisis-management" attitude and pressure to solve the organizational problems without delay. It also showed that in spite of their relatively small population bases and limited experiences, the local authorities, when properly motivated, can be effective in finding innovative solutions.

This law differed from all previous legislation in health and related fields. Typical of the previous "generation" of laws were normative regulations that mandated the number of personnel that had to be taken into account when the central authority paid its share of the costs. Such norms and details become obsolete in a relatively short time because it is not feasible to enact continuous small amendments to legislation. Because of such experiences, the law contained the explicit statement that it was only a framework for future actions. It indicated the direction in which development was to proceed and outlined the organizational configuration. The only detailed clauses related to the sharing of responsibilities and financial arrangements. The introduction of a formalized planning mechanism made possible the process of developing the organizational structure as well as the content of other functional aspects of primary care.

This legislation can be considered an innovation. At the conceptual level it can be perceived as a method of introducing a less rigid administrative "climate" that can facilitate a more progressive and innovative solution both now and in the future. It reflects a compromise between central and local administrative interests. The most important aspects of the legislation are summarized in the five points listed below. Each point represents innovative aspects that will be discussed subsequently.

1. The health center as the functional unit
2. A broader concept of primary-care functions
3. A suitable basis for population
4. Purposeful administration at the local level
5. The introduction of a formal planning mechanism

The Health Center as Functional Solution

The term *health center* has different meanings. In Finland it does not refer to a special building or to a department but to a *local organization that provides primary care or primary health services for the whole population* living inside known boundaries. In this respect the law is strict; it specifies that the local authority must develop, alone or together with other authorities, such a service unit. From the numerous theoretically possible organizational configurations that could have been selected the health center was chosen as a relatively strong, autonomous organization.

It would have been possible to link the health centers to regional, specialist-level hospitals. Under that arrangement, the centers would have functioned as outposts of polyclinics or outpatient departments of hospitals. That configuration would have eroded the interface between primary and secondary services, but, on the other hand, it might have introduced into the primary services the values, norms, and attitudes prevailing among inpatient care providers in specialist-level hospitals. It might have invalidated the objective of forming a health center especially oriented toward preventive care, such as screening and health education, by transforming it into a unit providing home care for chronic and minor illnesses, and so on, which usually do not occupy central positions in the hierarchy of hospital care.

During the developmental phase, it was decided to introduce the primary health services as an autonomous "system" with its own interests. Autonomy would make possible the formulation of local investment and manpower policies not subject to the control of strong interest groups favoring the further development of hospital services at the regional level. Thus it was envisioned that the problem of effecting an optimal balance among the various service sectors could be resolved.

The establishment of administrative boundaries between service subsystems usually produces some functional difficulties. But in this case, the integration of all existing local services into one administrative entity—the health center—abolished many jurisdictional problems. Nevertheless, some difficulties in effecting connections between the health centers and the regional hospital exist. Shortcomings have been observed in the level of cooperation achieved by the local services for health and for social welfare. The standard recommendation to solve such problems is general integration. Finland has been relatively cautious in adopting that strategy because, in practical terms, integration means that the resulting organization will be bigger and more complex. Furthermore, integration may introduce managerial problems, especially if it produces an imbalance between the values and the objectives of the organization. This kind of "cure" may be more harmful than the original problem that can often be solved by applying more specific remedies.

The New Concept of the Functions of Primary Care

There are interrelationships between basic societal goals and the actual functioning of the system. Goals are strategic in character and can be made operational by translating them into specific sets of objectives, preferably cast in quantitative terms. At least implicitly, objectives form a basis for selecting specified tasks or functions to be performed. The tasks determine the composition of the teams of health-care professionals within the units and influence the breadth of the facilities required.

Establishing health centers as the basic organizational solution did not introduce changes of such great magnitude that the goals or objectives could be labeled revolutionary. The services that were functioning on the basis of fragmented legislation could have been continued. The list of suggested activities revealed traditional thinking. It was not intended to be complete but to serve as a set of guidelines. In this respect, the law was well suited to serve as a framework, the content of which was to be determined by annual plans. This stipulation not only introduced the degree of flexibility required, especially in relation to functions, but to a marked extent made possible the restructuring of organizational operations.

In other words, it can be said that to the goals of primary health services was added the notion of *dynamic development*—not the achievement of a set of fixed objectives. The other goal that was especially stressed was *comprehensiveness*. These goals influenced the formulation of plans by focusing the planners' attention on the entire range of services. Related to the goal of comprehensiveness is the principle of *continuity*, which means that there must always be some unit that has direct responsibility for coordinating care, for example, rehabilitation and aftercare at home.

The Population Basis and Local Administration

The size of the population to be served by health centers is determined by the fact that population density is low, which means that basic services have to be provided in neighborhoods as well as in larger population centers. From the operational point of view, services that require more advanced technology or skills are critical. Such investments are justified at the primary level only if the entire range of resources can be used. Examples include X-ray and laboratory services, which are justified only if the catchment area is either large enough (35,000–50,000 inhabitants) or there are other needs to be served.

In Finland the second criterion served as the justification for the system that was adopted. Accordingly, it was decided that the health center should also have a ward of 30 beds for the acutely ill and about 60 beds for chronically ill patients. This arrangement justifies small catchment areas—about 10,000 to 15,000 inhabitants—for health centers. Another natural indicator of correct size is the required team configuration that should guarantee the continuity of service and at the same time take into account working hours and other comparable realities. When the legislation was enacted, there were about 500 local authorities, and of these, one-third had fewer than 5,000 inhabitants. It would have been possible—at least in theory—to introduce legislation that would have established norms for the smallest size of local authority. In practice, integrating local authority areas would have been complicated and time consuming because communal autonomy is highly valued. In order to organize primary health services on the basis of population, a much less dramatic innovation was required: cooperative action on the part of proximate local authorities. Opposition to cooperative action is not rational, and this objective was achieved without great difficulty.

The clauses in the law were formulated to give the local authority freedom to select its partner(s). But the law states that if there exist "special reasons," the cabinet can make cooperation obligatory. In approximately two years, the country was served by 218 health centers, of which 106 formed one and 112 two or more local authorities. Only in a few exceptional cases was the cabinet asked to decide how cooperation should be organized.

For about one hundred years there has been in each local authority area a local health board, whose members are elected by the local representative council. The law divided the health board into two sections, the first to be devoted to sanitary control and the second to the management of local health services. In Finland, no *ex officio* members serve on any politically responsible board, and this principle was applied in the case of the health board. The salaried medical officers have the right (or the obligation) to make proposals and function as experts, but they cannot participate in decision making.

This aspect of organizational development was not difficult to accomplish because the new configuration followed the general pattern and conformed to the technical situation. Even the requirement that cooperating local authorities establish a jointly nominated board of health was not perceived as a major problem.

Introduction of the Planning System

The ultimate goal of the "great leap" in organizational structure, framework, legislation, and so on was to make possible dynamic but rational development. Inevitably this development will be reflected not only in the volume of budgetary expenditures but also in procedures related to the formulation and the implementation of local and national budgets. With some exaggeration it can be said that the basic innovation involved the introduction of program budgeting in the health field. Traditional budgeting procedures stress fiscal and legal aspects, not executive or managerial flexibility and efficiency that are vital to rapid innovative development. Traditional budgeting focuses attention on resource inputs by type, but the resulting fragmentation makes it difficult to render coordinated decisions concerning strategic resource allocations. The solution to these problems in Finland was the adoption of a planning-programming-budgeting system (PPBS). The planning process was constructed so that local and central plans would be complementary parts of the same process. Inasmuch as small legislative details can be decisive in the implementation of principles, there is reason to focus attention on two such details. One is the subsidizing procedure. The law follows the traditional Finnish pattern: The primary responsible actors are local authorities, and the acceptable expenses are subsidized by the central government. At present, subsidies range from 39 to 70 percent. The percentages are based on yearly ratings of taxable incomes earned in each local authority. The objective is to encourage activity on the part of representatives from the economically less developed parts of the country.

Subsidies are *conditional*, that is, they are to be paid only for acceptable activities. In the past, such judgments were usually deferred, and only technical criteria were employed in the process of evaluation. The new law introduced the principle that *an approved plan gives to the local authority the right to obtain central governmental subsidies.* This stipulation makes the plans important documents and gives the central government considerable scope for guidance without dictating what the local authorities should do and unduly limiting their autonomy.

Another clause that deserves attention is the requirement that *the central authority must approve the plan in toto—not in part.* This stipulation means that a local authority could lose all subsidies if the plan does not conform to the norms or is considered inappropriate. If the local authorities and the central government representatives (the National Board of Health) cannot agree on the content of the local plan, the cabinet makes the decision. In practice, the bargaining process nearly always produces a solution that is acceptable to all parties concerned.

These two aspects make coordinated planning important and yield benefits when the local authority is active but give to the central authority a strong role in allocating resources as well as in influencing the content of individual programs. The planning horizon extends five years beyond the year covered by traditional one-year budgets. A corrected plan is composed every year at all levels.

In a parliamentary form of government such as Finland's, long-term budgeting is complicated because no cabinet can make binding decisions for a longer term than the budget period, which is usually one year. Parliament can enact laws that are valid at least until the next election, but because of the minority clauses, such laws are not feasible alternatives. In Finland, the problem was solved by letting the cabinet—not the parliament—endorse financial statements pertaining to the plan. The document is made public, and the political opposition can accordingly voice reservations about its content. Reservations can be put into effect if/when the cabinet is reconstituted—a common phenomenon in Finland. There are not very marked differences in the health policies advocated by the political parties, and cabinet proposals concerning the allocation of resources have often been realized in spite of changes in its composition.

The Principles of PPBS

There is no need to discuss the technical details of PPBS.[7] The basic principle involves formulating a plan for a medium-term period, quantifying programs when appropriate, and stating as explicitly as possible the value judgments involved. The primary tool for evaluating programs and controlling actions is the budget, which allocates money for functions. The first step in program budgeting is the division of activities into "mission-oriented" building blocks called program elements. Such elements incorporate definable tasks and are comprised of persons, facilities, material, and so on. Examples of program elements in primary care are maternity health, vaccination, transportation for the sick, home visiting, and so on. The elements are assembled in "major programs" defined by mission or objective. Examples are MCH services, the fight against infectious diseases, long-term care, and so on. Such major programs contain closely related elements that should be considered manifestations of the basic missions or goals of the service sector. The missions of examples previously cited can be summarized in the following terms:

improving the health of the next generation
abolishing the risk of contagious diseases
caring for the chronically ill

The previous presentation stresses budgetary aspects, but this kind of planning process can be applied in principle to any managerial problem. Program budgeting requires the close interaction of the operating, analytical, and decision-making segments of an organization. It often requires focusing attention on problems that go far beyond the decision situation as initially perceived. In a recent policy statement entitled "Blueprint for Health for All," the director-general of the WHO[8] strongly recommended this kind of planning system as a mechanism for health development. "Programme Budgeting at the Country Level—A Golden Opportunity" was one of the headings of the presentation. Finland's experiences, gained during the two years since the PPBS modification was applied, definitely supports this statement.

F. EVALUATIVE CONCLUSIONS

Techniques of Change

The framework legislation and the built-in planning mechanism for dynamic development are, of course, techniques for change. Decisive for overall success is the proper balance between the solid frame and flexibility in planning developmental actions. Only a framework for future activities was devised—the actual functions would be defined on the basis of the built-in mechanism of continuous planning. Prevailing societal values, such as comprehensiveness, equity, and continuity, should inform the planning process to such an extent that the organizational configuration and functions develop in a purposeful direction. Health is well suited to such an approach because there is no great disagreement among social strata or political parties about basic values and principles. This relative consensus was one of the prerequisites of success.

Formal authorization is, of course, one prerequisite of PPBS, but equally important is the relation between active cooperation and direct rewards. This relationship is especially important when numerous small autonomous units—local authorities—function in a cooperative manner with the central government. The plans of local authorities should form a national program so that relevant expenditures can be taken into account in the national budget. The most important "power elements" in the past, elements that have been incorporated into the new arrangements, were state subsidies. In the past they were granted "if the cost of the work done was acceptable." The new legislation grants subsidies "if they [local authorities] follow an accepted plan."

Central government subsidies could be withheld, at least in theory, if the proposed innovative actions are rejected. This rejection would make financially unbearable the burden on local authorities and would most likely influence the election of the next communal council. Undeniably, the planning process has limited to some extent the autonomy of local authorities, but this limitation has been imposed to the smallest possible extent and has been offset by other benefits, for example, the longer planning horizon and the development of primary health services. The opinion of the "man on the street" so strongly favors the innovation that the local council would have to present very special reasons for being uncooperative and delaying development.

Elementary aspects of innovative policy relate to systematic education, guidance, the dissemination of information, and so on. The central authority functioned for a few months in a way that closely resembled a military headquarters. Under the coordinating group there were three "strategic" working groups (for legal problems, for work descriptions, and for economic questions) and numerous expert groups that defined technical tasks. The prime movers were a few leading administrators who took full managerial responsibility for the process.

Adopters and Users

Involved in this chain of events were numerous adopters. First were members of parliament who transformed the principles into legislative measures. Other adopters were the national unions of local authorities that influenced the attitudes of their members. They were well represented in the working groups. In theory, the electors of the local council were adopters. In practice, the local councils were interested in taking advantage of the opportunity to develop health services.

Impact and Experiences

In a brief time, a network of functioning health centers was constructed from elements that already existed. The impact on the volume of services and functions was negative during the phase of organizational restructuring, but in a relatively short period of time, the volume of output increased. The same can be said of the other outputs mentioned in Paragraph C.

The planned innovation produced positive side effects. Perhaps the most valuable long-term impact will be reflected in the behavior and the attitudes of decision makers functioning at different levels. The basic elements of the innovation are not formal plans or informational aspects but positive attitudes that are manifest in adapting the system to changing environmental and internal forces. In this respect, the "dramatized" implementation of "planning" provided basic training and experience in "modern management." It seems that this impact will endure and that the resulting organizational configuration will continue to support its further development.

The attitude reflected in this paper is that of an insider working in the central government. Accordingly, some bias may be apparent. The outsiders–for example, the local authorities–criticized, quite justifiably, the short implementation period. The innovation changed the accustomed roles and salary systems of some personnel groups. To some extent, criticism could have been avoided if due attention had been given to such problems. Local authorities were not happy when they were obliged to fill in forms that sometimes required quantitative information that did not exist. This part of the problem was solved easily, but the argument is voiced continuously, year after year.

The most difficult problem seems to be that most adopters and users have not developed balanced views of the key issues of innovations. Program budgeting, which requires the repeated formulation of plans, is often presented as a "nuisance." This contention could have been avoided if more attention had been devoted to theoretical issues and principles. To a marked extent, budgeting problems are unavoidable especially when economic stagnation limits progress. There must be someone who can be blamed, and a new budgeting procedure serves as a surrogate for such a purpose. Coping with sudden economic changes in the absence of continuously revised forecasts is difficult both for those who are responsible for the national economy as well as for national and local policymakers in the health field.

G. SUMMARY

In this chapter the focus of interest centers on organizational development, especially the introduction of planned changes. The innovation involved an organizational configuration that supports continuous development and makes central control possible but decentralizes decision-making processes as much as possible. What is the best solution, what can be achieved, and how should adopters and users behave are questions that relate to societal values, to the environment in which the service system functions, and to the actors and their motivations. In this chapter the point of view is that of the national authorities.

This case study is based on a real experiment in which the theoretical aspects of introducing innovations were not considered. But even an impressionistic evaluation suggests that most of the principles were applied and conduced to the extensive reorganization that occurred. The planned changes were introduced in a much shorter time than is usually considered realistic. Introducing innovations, for example, organizational restructuring, seems to be a useful technique that should become part of the armament of planners in the social-service sector.

REFERENCES

1. WHO. *Organizational Study on Methods of Promoting the Development of Basic Health Services.* Geneva: WHO Off. Records no. 206, 1973.
2. WHO. *Development of Health Programme Evaluation.* Thirty-first World Health Assembly, A 31/10. Geneva, 1978.
3. OECD. *Policies for Innovation in the Service Sector.* Paris, 1977.
4. Hakkarainen, A. *Introducing Primary Health Services on a Nationwide Scale* (DSTI/SPR/75.60/22B). Ref. OECD. Policies of Innovation . . . , 1977.
5. Puro, Kari. *Our Health* (Kansanterveytemme). H.S. 20, 22, and 25, October 1971 (About six newspaper pages in Finnish).
6. Lindblom, C. E. "The Science of 'Muddling Through.' " *Publ. Adm. Rev.* 1959: 19:79–99.
7. Novick, D., and Euthoven, A. "Long-Range Planning Through Program Budgeting." In *Perspectives of Planning.* Ed. E. Jantsch. Paris: OECD, 1969 (no. 24421), pp. 254–283.
8. Mahler, H. Blueprint for Health for All. *WHO Chronicle.* 1977: 31:491–498.

Chapter 14

National Health Initiatives and Local Health-Insurance Carriers: The Case of the Federal Republic of Germany

Christa Altenstetter

INTRODUCTION

German and English-speaking scholars in different fields of social science in recent years have paid considerable attention to the economics and the politics of the national health-insurance program (GKV) and the formulation of other health programs in the Federal Republic of Germany. Even though this growing literature has closed gaps in knowledge about German health-care policy and the delivery system, important areas remain unresearched. Mapping the importance of organizations that implement health programs is one area that scholars have hardly pursued. The institutions that intervene in the implementation of the national health-insurance program—the sickness funds—is another. Although their roles as bargainers with providers have changed over the years, giving them less influence today than they had in the past, citizens' direct or indirect contact with the funds is as important, inevitable, and recurring as that with the German IRS.

National provisions outline fairly comprehensively conditions of membership, entitlement, coverage, and related matters. They apply nationwide to all actors in the German health-care delivery system as well as to all political and organizational actors in the national polity at large. From the perspective of individuals, no service or cash payments can be received nor can time periods be calculated toward benefits payable at retirement without proper registration with a sickness fund. Although the first day of work secures and activates legal entitlement, registration with a sickness fund provides tangible and concrete entry to the health-care system and to the benefits and protection that the German welfare state has granted over the decades. Sickness funds collect not only the contributions to the public health insurance program but also to three German social insurance programs (retirement, disability, and unemployment). National provisions require all employers to register with the sickness fund their employees and those whom national stipulations single out as mandatory or voluntary members and liable for payments to these social insurance programs. Typically, national provisions on income ceilings determine membership. Dependents become entitled to receive services and benefits through the proper registration of the breadwinner only. Sickness funds administer other national or state programs, such as the maternity allowance program, the health insurance program for students, assistance programs for prisoners, and disabled veterans, their widows, and orphans, and accident insurance, to mention only a few.

Few would debate the fact that the public health-insurance program was among the most important innovations in social policy and institutional developments in the nineteenth century. Its impact on developments in the search for a proper vehicle to administer health and income programs in neighboring and distant countries is widely documented. The objectives of the program were to provide coverage and benefits as well as income during sickness, at first, to the bottom income layer of the German population. Today coverage extends to about 90 percent of the German population. Since its inception, the program has constituted the centerpiece of German health and social policy and is certain to remain so, irrespective of innovations that the federal legislature may mandate in the existing program, in administrative and financing procedures, or in organizational arrangements for the delivery of services.

In terms of institutional innovations, the model of governance that was adopted for the administration of the public-health insurance program in the nineteenth century in Germany was extended to all social-insurance carriers, albeit with some modifications. The development of labor-management organizations represented the triumph of a political principle advocated by the labor movement. The model of self-governance (*Selbstverwaltung*) remains sacrosanct today for most political groups, although they may advance different reasons to defend it. Despite its long history and the political as well as the institutional significance of self-governance, we know more about the normative postulates of the principle than about its functioning in general sickness funds. This contribution sheds some light on the typical governance structure of a general sickness fund (AOK), the decision makers involved, and their roles and responsibilities.

First, we discuss some electoral and constitutional issues of self-governance and then present the main divisions and allocations of responsibilities to the major decision makers of a sickness fund. A description of the actual exercise of these responsibilities constitutes the main part of this contribution, followed by concluding comments and a summary.

We rely heavily on documentation published by general sickness funds and on information provided by local officials in six general sickness funds who were interviewed during the months of September and December 1978. The funds visited were those of Düsseldorf, Siegerland-Wittgenstein, and Hochsauerlandkreis in North-Rhine Westfalia and Munich, Weiden, and Amberg in Bavaria. The funds are located in urban and rural areas that are part of a larger study on implementing national health programs in the Federal Republic of Germany. Because of the confidential nature of the subject matter, some materials and sources of personal interviews are not identified. The reports of the sickness funds are listed in the bibliography.

GOVERNANCE

The governance structure of general sickness funds is similar to that of other social-insurance carriers. Since the nineteenth century realization of the concept of self-governance has required the existence of two separate decision-making bodies. The assembly "legislates" and the governing board "executes." Today national provisions outline requirements for equal representation of the insured population and business interests as well as procedures governing their election. In practice, representation of the insured population is limited to working people through trade union representatives. In the nineteenth century, workers had greater formal representation than they have today: a two-thirds majority of workers' representatives on the assembly and on the board faced a one-third minority of business representatives. In 1934 Selbstverwaltung was abolished. Instead of a committee, a council (*Beirat*) was heard on a few topics. The role of the board was reduced. Executive directors controlled the sickness funds. Legislation in 1952 reinstalled Selbstverwaltung but made a major change: half the members on the assembly and on the board are now from trade unions.

Much has been written in support of continuing this model of equal representation and governance for the administration of sickness funds.[1]

From the perspective of a typical member of a sickness fund, however, one may raise a question about the adequacy of representation of all insured persons. The composition of the membership is drastically different today from what it was in the nineteenth century. Members of the labor force were the only insured population group then, whereas today they constitute about half the typical membership of a fund. (True, they continue to be the most important financial contributors.) Homemakers and dependent children, retired persons, students, and other groups constitute the other half.

In his examination of the development of Selbstverwaltung, Tennstedt points to the considerable gap that has historically existed between the claim for and the reality of workers' representation vis-à-vis management. According to him, two phases had to be completed before workers' influence could be exerted in the governance of sickness funds. He distinguishes three distinct phases of development in the period from 1883 to 1918. During the first phase, the state supervisory agencies created the general sickness funds and assumed responsibility for administering and controlling them. During the second phase, employers' representatives began to operate and exercise influence over decision making in the funds. Only in the third phase did freely organized workers begin to serve in the general assemblies and on the boards.

Most of the literature on self-governance stresses the organizational autonomy of local sickness funds. Indeed, funds are quasi-public administrative entities separate from public administration. They are authorized to set law in statutes and through guidelines. They also determine what administrative procedures must be followed in carrying out their program responsibilities. Technically and legally, the characterization of organizational autonomy is correct; but it obscures the reality that the law narrowly and comprehensively prescribes what sickness funds can or must do, how they do what they can or must do, and for what aspects of their activities and under what circumstances they are accountable to what segment of government.[2] Federal and state agencies have retained considerable supervisory authority over important responsibilities. This authority is defined and has been primarily invoked to determine whether decisions and actions taken by the assembly and the board conform to federal and state laws and regulations. Supervisory authority is formidable when it is used as an instrument of government to control local sickness funds. This instrument includes supervisory control over four important "autonomous" responsibilities of local sickness funds. Funds are responsible for:

a. developing and passing their own statutes or constitution, so to speak;

b. formulating work provisions (*Dienstordnung*);
c. setting contribution rates to balance their budgets in line with federal provisions; and
d. formulating rules of behavior with respect to health regulations (*Krankenordnung*).

In addition to these "autonomous" responsibilities, health-insurance carriers administer "delegated" responsibilities, for example, the administration of social-insurance programs (retirement, unemployment, and disability) as well as other social programs.

A clue to the actual meaning of organizational autonomy and independence in decision making lies in the legal phrase that permits the government to influence and interfere with the internal affairs of health-insurance carriers only through legislation. The federal government—especially in the areas of health and social policies—and the states—especially in the areas of administration and supervision as well as employment—have not refrained from legislating responsibilities for the funds, thereby undermining organizational and, to a certain extent, financial autonomy. Numerous constraints have been imposed on the funds. Regulations concerning how and for whom funds must spend their resources emanate from program stipulations in the public health-insurance program as well as from provisions in numerous other social programs that local sickness funds administer for other public agencies. Recommendations by the National Association of Physicians and Sickness Funds (*Bundesausschuss der Ärzte und Krankenkassen*), for example, which are usually endorsed by state associations, interfere with internal decision-making processes. The courts have limited the funds in their decision making through the issuance of an increasing number of rulings on health insurance and other social-insurance programs.

Indeed, we may ask what good formal autonomy is when external political and administrative actors meticulously and comprehensively define the basic parameters of responsibilities and rules to be obeyed by the staff and the governing bodies of an organization. What good is organizational autonomy, when an organization cannot decide the responsibilities it wants to engage in? Sickness funds can engage only in program activities that legislation assigns them. Control over one's organizational resources usually indicates independence, but in the case of sickness funds, organizational resources and capacities are subject to considerable direct and indirect influence exerted by external controllers.

Despite the extensive and growing government influence over local sickness funds and their operations, recent reforms and provisions concerning the self-governance of social-insurance carriers reinforce the political mandate and the thrust of the objectives of health and social-insurance administration developed in the course of one hundred years.[3] More recent political goals adressed by the reforms include strengthening the possibilities of controlling the financial and the organizational capacities of sickness funds and influencing the availability and the distribution of services to those who are entitled or who need to receive them. However, in light of the restrictions imposed on sickness funds by national policy, there seems to be a gap between what self-governance ought to do and what it can do in day-to-day operations. Elections are an important instrument, but legal prescriptions seem to exert considerable influence on the actions of sickness funds.

The literature has addressed the importance of social elections to social-insurance carriers primarily from a normative perspective and secondarily from an empirical one.[4] To the extent that researchers are interested in the actual results of elections, they are usually concerned with elections to the national or regional organizations. Comparative analyses of elections in individual funds and of different participation rates as well as possible explanations of why elections differ regionally and from fund to fund are nonexistent. Rates of electoral participation are said to oscillate between a high of 40 to 30 percent and a low of around 20 percent. Although social elections may cause embarrassment because of the gap between claims and realities, they continue to be very important in national and regional politics, as the elections in the summer of 1980 demonstrated. True elections of independent candidates have never occurred in any of the funds. Prior to elections, business and trade union representatives approve of one list of candidates, adhering to the requirement of proportional representation. Being listed guarantees a candidate's election.

In the hierarchy of binding rules that impinge on fund governance, statutes are less significant than federal and state laws, federal and state regulations, and court rulings. Statutes outline basic governance structures of and details about local operations. Laws provide for a formal division of authority and responsibilities between self-governing bodies and management. But they also authorize the issuance of statutes that may provide more details about the allocation of responsibilities. Thus the authority to develop statutes and to amend them in case of need is one important responsibility of fund decision makers.

Analyses of statutes yields these observations: Statutes vary in comprehensiveness and format, including the order in which individual provisions and major chapter headings are presented. But by and large, they follow the model of statutes recommended by federal policymakers. Some funds reprint legal provisions as well as legal jargon. Others reformulate and rephrase legal provisions into laymen's language. Sometimes comprehensiveness or brevity is a reflection of the age of the statute or the date on which it was amended. Statutes of the AOK München, the largest sickness fund interviewed, are representative of other statutes.[5] They illustrate more vividly and impressively than any legal or political treatise could that little genuine and independent decision-making authority obtains in self-governing institutions.

To avoid the problem of having to reprint statutes each time laws and program stipulations change, the AOK München, like other funds, prints statutes in three colors. White pages indicate areas of local or "autonomous" decision making by the fund; pink pages list provisions set by the federal legislature; and yellow pages indicate federal provisions covering the wage-continuation program.

To estimate the proportion of fund decision making to federal decision making, I counted the number of pages and the relative space devoted to autonomous fund policymaking and federal policymaking. Of a total of about eighty-nine pages of small print, about forty-three white pages indicate a surprisingly important area of decision-making responsibility left to the board and to the assembly and, to a lesser extent, to the administration. But a spot check of individual topics revealed a different picture, which indicates the relative distribution of decision making between federal legislators and fund decision makers. For example, in checking statutory provisions on the governance of the AOK München, it was found that four main items consisting of a short sentence each were supplemented by a total of nine pages of federal provisions with nine major headings. Each heading consists mostly of a couple of sentences each. For one page of statutory provisions about the responsibilities of the board, there are two pages of federal provisions detailing what the board is supposed to do. For one sentence setting forth the authority of the executive director, there is one full page of federal provisions.

The authority of the AOK München to decide benefits and services is outlined on one page. Federal stipulations cover two pages. The authority to decide benefits over and above the nationally mandated level is outlined on half a page, whereas four pages of legal text define federal details covering additional benefits (*Mehrleistung*). Finally, there are no white pages on the wage-continuation program; instead, four pages of federal provisions outline what the funds are to do. We could continue indefinitely what some may consider an inappropriate approach to the identification of the extent of the fund's autonomous decision making. The point is clearly made, however: important policy and administrative matters are contained in the pink pages, whereas the content of the white pages is less significant.

We ventured one guess about which kind of fund would delineate areas of responsibilities between political decision makers and management.

We assumed that the larger the fund, the more specific this assignment of responsibility would be. In several instances, the reverse was true. Small funds were more restrictive concerning the authority of management vis-à-vis the assembly and the board than were large funds. Should we conclude that self-governance in small funds is politically more alive? Are the boards of small funds more interested than those of large funds in the well-being of the organization? Or cannot large funds afford to have weak managers who need to refer to the boards—which meet once per month at a maximum—for approval of major and minor decisions? Have not the statutes of some funds been revised recently? We cannot answer these questions, but the findings point to the importance of different environments in devising formal tools for operating sickness funds.

Decision Makers

Figure 14.1 outlines the major decision makers (or *Organe der Krankenkassen*) in a fund and identifies the electoral and operational linkages between them. The members of the board and the assembly, in addition to the executive director, are singled out as the most important decision makers. However, little is known about the functions of additional actors in each sickness fund. The following range of decision makers and actors typically influences decision making in a fund:

The board as collective actor
- The Chairman of the Board
- The Deputy of the Board
- The committees of the board
- Individual board members

The assembly as collective actor
- Assembly members
- The Chairman of the Assembly
- The Deputy of the Assembly
- The committees of the assembly

Management
- The Executive Director
- The Deputy Executive Director
- The administration of the Sickness Fund and Staff

Eldermen or spokesmen of the membership of the fund
Trustees of business

National provisions pertaining to the self-governance of social-insurance carriers provide for detailed procedures about how to convene meetings, how to take votes at meetings, how to organize and hold elec-

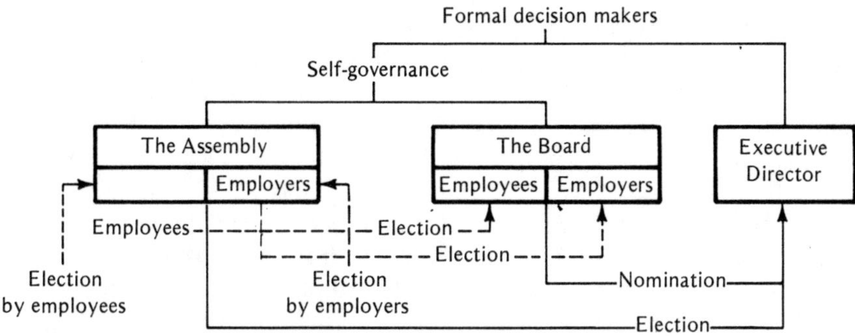

Source: "Fortbildung: Thema: Die Selbstverwaltung in der gesetzlichen Krankenversicherung," *Soziale Krankenversicherung*, 8 (1979), p. 317.

Figure 14.1. Major decision makers in a fund.

tions to the assembly and the board, and related matters. Even the number of representatives from the two political constituencies on the board and the assembly is prescribed. According to the statutes, each fund must determine the number of assembly and board members as a function of membership size. Table 14.1, illustrating the proportion of assembly to board members, indicates this mandated symmetry. As the table indicates, the assembly as the "legislature" is from three to four times the size of the board as the "executive."

Table 14.1. Proportion of Assembly Members to Board Members, and Number of Business and Trade Union Representatives on Each

Fund	*Board*	*Assembly*	*Members*
AOK München	7:7	30:30	493,532
AOK Düsseldorf	6:6	20:20	157,106
AOK Amberg	6:6	18:18	66,012
AOK Weiden	5:5	15:15	40,113
AOK Hochsauerlandkreis[a]	6:6	24:24	82,251
AOK Siegerland-Wittgenstein[a]	5:5	18:18	64,155

Source: Statutes of individual sickness funds and Bundesverband der Ortskrankenkassen, *Statistik der Ortskrankenkassen 1976.*

Note: For an interim period the AOK Hochsauerlandkreis will have a twenty-six-member board and a seventy-two-member assembly, and the AOK Siegerland-Wittgenstein will have an eighteen-member board and a sixty-member assembly.

[a] The figures for the two funds are for the new board and assembly starting in 1980. From several separate funds each fund was merged into a larger fund.

The Assembly and Its Responsibilities. The assembly passes its own bylaws (*Geschäftsordnung*) and elects representatives to the three institutions—the assembly, the board, and management—which constitute the formal decision makers. The assembly elects the chairman of the assembly and his deputy as well as members to the governing board and the deputies. Since 1977 the assembly has elected the executive director on the advice of the board. In terms of financial control, the assembly approves the budget of the preceding year and authorizes the budget for the coming year. On the advice of the board, the assembly decides remuneration for members of the self-governing bodies. All members who serve in the assembly or on the board are unpaid, but on the board's advice, the assembly decides what remuneration the representatives will receive for travel and subsidy allowance. Changes in statutes as well as fund policy are decided by the assembly. In addition, the assembly must formally approve contracts with providers, voluntary agreements with other sickness funds, and joining or leaving an association. It also formulates the rules on health behavior (*Krankenordnung*) for patients and the sanctions imposed on a fund member if he or she disregards them.[6] Although the health regulations were important enforcement instruments for funds and were widely used in previous decades, they are of minor significance today.

To implement the health insurance program and, more significantly, other social-security programs or parts thereof, funds are required to set up registration (*Meldestellen*) and payment (*Zahlstellen*) offices. The assembly makes the formal decision to establish them or to close them. Fund members and business firms are entitled to complain about and appeal decisions of the fund; the assembly legislates provisions on how to do so. Therefore, each fund has a complaint service (*Widerspruchstelle*). It is administered separately from the management of the fund by two voluntary officials who are unpaid and elected by the assembly on the basis of equal representation. Finally, each fund runs an assembly-approved appeals service (*Einspruchstelle*).

Even though the formulation of work provisions (*Dienstordnung*) is one of the board's prerogatives, the assembly must ratify them. Transfers of assets and liabilities that may result from a merger or a separation of funds require the approval of the assembly. The assembly also has the formal authority to set up hospitals and convalescent homes. In practice, hospital ownership by the funds is the exception rather than the rule. But such large funds as Düsseldorf and München own and run their own facilities. For example, the AOK Düsseldorf runs a dental clinic and several optical shops, and the AOK München has convalescent homes in the mountains. Small funds usually do not own facilities. Some funds add other responsibilities to their statutes, which the assembly can approve.

For example, the statutes of two funds provide for assembly approval of the bylaws of the board, and three funds require assembly approval for establishing and closing fund-owned and fund-operated facilities.

The Board and Its Responsibilities. Like the assembly, the board elects the deputy chairman and the chairman. The chairman is assigned special responsibilities under the law. The chairman and the deputy do not represent the same constituency: one represents trade union interests and the other represents business interests. To safeguard the chair from being monopolized by one group, the chair rotates each year. Rotation also occurs in the chair of the assembly.

As a collective body, the board is endowed with special legal and administrative responsibilities. The more important ones are prescribed by law and the remaining ones by statutes. For example, the board releases members of the board and the assembly from their official responsibilities at the completion of their terms. In extreme cases the board may dismiss a member for violating the code and provisions of responsibilities of representatives of the fund. The board must make certain that successors to elected members and their deputies who resign or whose terms of office have expired are elected properly.

Until the enactment of the reforms of 1977, the board had exclusive authority to select, nominate, and appoint the executive director and his deputy without assembly approval. The 1977 reforms require that candidates who are nominated by the board must be elected by the assembly. In theory, the new provision limits the board's authority. In practice, this provision may mean only that board members might have to lobby for their candidates among assembly members; the chairman and the deputy—each of whom represents a different constituency—enjoy the confidence of their respective followers in the assembly. Consequently, they constitute the natural access and liaison points. The board develops and approves its own bylaws. According to some statutes, bylaws must be approved by the assembly. As the main governing body, the board is responsible for formulating day-to-day policy and management. Because of this responsibility, relations between the board and management are closer—and contact between them more frequent—than those between management and the assembly.

Meetings of the assembly usually take place twice a year for budget authorization for the next year in November, and for approval of the budget for the past year in June. In contrast, the board, on which the executive director serves in an advisory capacity, usually meets once per month in the large funds and about three to four times per year in smaller funds. Not all areas of activities and responsibilities undertaken by the executive director and management are prescribed and outlined by law. In cases in which a program allows for some interpretation and discretion, the board can pass guidelines. These guidelines are binding on top management and the administration of the fund. Although the guidelines are supposed to assist management in decision making, they function to curb management's authority to pursue a policy that may not have the endorsement of the board.

Usually board guidelines inform such areas as the following:

employment and staff policy;
cash-benefit allowances for househelpers and house health care;
rehabilitation subsidies;
travel allowances for visits to providers if the fund has ordered such a visit;
hardship cases resulting from the 1977 law on cost containment; and
prevention.

Conflicts with policymakers at state and federal levels occur quite often in areas for which the board has sole authority to take initiatives and decide policy. The local funds seem to be caught between what they can afford to pay and what their national counterparts ask them to do for ideological and political reasons. For example, the 1977 national recommendation on hardship cases suggested a monthly income of DM 3000 as the criterion for eligibility for benefits under the program. In some cases this income ceiling meant that almost 80 or 90 percent of a fund's population would become eligible, which in turn meant additional financial burdens for the fund. About 50 percent of local funds are said to have disregarded the federal recommendation and set a much lower income ceiling. Tensions between local funds on the one hand and between state and federal associations on the other were mentioned repeatedly, but little systematic information about who won and who lost is available. Rehabilitation and prevention apparently continue to be subject to some influence of the board.

The same officials formulate national recommendations. Officials of state associations (LdO) sit on the board of the national association (BdO). From the local perspective, the national board can easily formulate and transmit national recommendations through state associations to the local funds for application. Although the national and state associations incur no financial responsibility, local sickness funds do, and they also incur additional work loads.

Personnel policy and employment guidelines are of particular importance not only for day-to-day management but also for the fund as employer. Formally the board formulates, approves, and, in case of need, amends work provisions (*Dienstordnung*). Like statutes and health regulations, for example, work provisions require the approval of the state supervisory agency. Formulating policy on employment and promotion in the Dienstordnung has often been cited as one of the remnants of important responsibilities over which the fund exercises autonomous decision making. But comprehensive and continuously changing national and state laws as well as collective-bargaining agreements take precedence over any provision that the board may formulate. In fact, the impact of national and state developments on manpower, wages, salaries, and fringe benefits is as far-reaching and restrictive on the funds as national provisions relating to health-services administration and financing that leave little room for local action (2. Gesetz zur Vereinheitlichung und Neuregelung des Besoldunngsrechts in Bund und Ländern). Why would funds oppose federal or state provisions that offer better job security, pay, and fringe benefits than those offered by a single local sickness fund? Higher pay and better fringe benefits affect the fund as employer in terms of higher outlays for personnel costs. Funds have no choice: they must follow national or state contracts, which affect about 50 percent of the staff in a sickness fund. The remaining 50 percent enjoy a status similar to that of civil service.

The board has formal authority to hire, fire, promote, and give notice to staff members as well as to approve applications for retirement. In the past, the board's authority to hire whom its members wanted must have been crucial. Today this responsibility amounts to little more than applying contractual agreements and effecting employment conditions negotiated elsewhere.

Some statutes specify the grades that require board approval for new staff members, whereas others apparently leave this decision to top management. The boards of all sickness funds must approve contracts for trainees. Loans, transfers of assets and liabilities, and the opening of a facility that is owned by the fund require the approval of the board as well as that of the assembly. In addition, board approval is necessary for expenditures that exceed the limit set for decision making by the executive director.

Negotiations with hospitals on daily service charges that sickness funds have to pay for hospitalized members are decentralized. Individual funds have more influence over those charges vis-à-vis the state association and the hospitals than over negotiations for fee-for-service reimbursements. In Bavaria the funds, with the assistance of the state association, negotiate hospital charges with each hospital in their service areas; daily hospital service charges are among the lowest in Germany. In contrast, negotiations in Northrhine Westfalia take place at the substate-regional level but not at the level of individual funds. Members from local funds, assisted by a representative from the respective state association (LdO), constitute the negotiating team (Einigungskommission) for the region. (For historical reasons, there are several separate regional teams for hospitals in the region of Northrhine and others for Westfalia. Prior to 1945, Northrhine and Westfalia were separate territories with strong historical traditions.) By and large, the service charges are higher there than they are in Bavaria. There is an apparent correlation between the kind of decision-making systems and the level of expenditures for hospitals. This relationship will be examined separately.

Although funds do not determine expenditures for medical and dental appliances, they have to abide by state contracts entered into with a wide range of medical providers and suppliers and nonmedical providers. In previous decades funds had more independence. In Bavaria, state contracts with medical drug suppliers have been operative since 1970, in Northrhine since 1970, and in Westfalia since 1972.[7] These contracts, which commit limited resources that constitute the total expenditures of a fund, serve an important economic function in the local economy. In some communities and regions, a general sickness fund may be the only insurance carrier that caters to the local and regional population. Consequently, the fund is a crucial source of revenues for local shops. Officials who were interviewed insisted on the significance of these direct relations with local shops and facilities. But, given these state contracts, the extent to which funds can negotiate their own conditions has not been clarified. Are opticians, specialist shoemakers, and related craftworkers considered suppliers to members of the fund simply because they are certified by the state? Or can a fund accept one shop and refuse to pay for material supplied by another? The approval and the acceptance of these contracts fall within the responsibility of the board as governing body.

A final group of responsibilities includes legal and contractual matters. First, the board has authority to delay, cancel, exempt, or negotiate compromises on contributions and other cash claims in cases that exceed the national income ceiling. The board must obtain the approval of a third party if this party has some financial claim. Second, the board must determine and assess a higher share of employers' contributions in special cases. Third, the board approves any agreement that provides rehabilitation services, operating services, and information centers for the handicapped.

Four kinds of special responsibilities are reserved to the chairman of the board: (1) ensuring that all decisions and actions taken by the staff of the fund conform to federal laws, statutes, and work provisions and taking disciplinary action against an employee if necessary; (2) authorizing nonroutine payments and compensation to the executive director; (3) voting on behalf of the fund as employer and requesting the nomination of candidates for election to the board and to the assembly; and (4) announcing the results of elections and indicating any change in the composition of the board and of the assembly. In short, the chairman is singled out not only in a legal-administrative capacity but also in a political capacity. Rotation in office on the part of the chairman and the deputy who both represent a different constituency is a natural and logical consequence of this political role.

HOW DYNAMIC OR STATIC IS SELF-GOVERNANCE?

The preceding sections described the formal responsibilities of the assembly and the board and indicated that self-governance is indeed alive. This section focuses on the exercise of these responsibilities. What parts do the board and the assembly and their various committees and subcommittees play in making decisions and setting priorities? What does information from the field reveal about self-governance? Is self-governance more a fiction than a reality?

The Assembly

On paper and by federal intention, the assembly of health-insurance funds, like those of other social-insurance carriers, appears to be a powerful elected body. It "legislates" policy for the fund and controls its manpower and financial and organizational resources. In particular, the assembly has authority to vote on the work provisions, the health regulations, and the statutes of the fund. The purpose of this research was to find out not only the scope of the assembly's de facto influence but also which responsibilities officials considered more important than others from the perspective of their own experience. No unanimity was expressed in evaluating certain responsibilities over others, and perceptions about the area or areas over which the assembly exercises the most influence ranged from the formal authority to approve the budget and set contribution rates to the authority to decide property matters, the recent authority to develop a job plan, and finally the authority to issue the work provisions and other stipulations. Set forth below are the paraphrased responses of interviewed officials:

> The possibility that the assembly may elect the wrong board can mean that the leadership of the fund may take the wrong direction. Without a good board not a single responsibility will work out. Consequently, I would consider the election of the board the primary task of the assembly. Of course, approval of the budget and the statutes is also important. But without a good or the right board nothing works.

Approval of the budget is the most important responsibility, and the budget is always approved.

Budget authorization, approval of the job plan, formulating and authorizing the health regulations, and approval of the work provisions for DO-Angestellte exhaust the list of responsibilities that the assembly exercises in giving binding instructions to management.

To decide on the statute is the most important authority of the assembly. Federal legislation limits this authority continuously and considerably. For this reason, differences between the funds are unimportant. The second most important responsibility is to control and authorize the budget. For this purpose the assembly usually meets in June and in December. The public supervisory agencies have recently attempted to gain access to the budgeting process of self-governing institutions. There are plans to adjust the provisions on budgeting for quasi-public, self-governing institutions to those of the governmental sector.

Collecting contributions, passing the statutes—which is almost equal in importance to concerns with contributions—and approving the work provisions are important responsibilities.

One cannot generalize about the meetings of the assembly. They differ from meeting to meeting. Of course, decisions about contribution rates and finances play an important role. Demands for more services and benefits give rise to discussions and tough confrontations between the two constituencies. Naturally, the new provision on the election of the executive director by the assembly means politicization.

One can speak of the assembly's loss of responsibilities. Self-governance of the general sickness funds is based on an ambivalence that is reflected in the different interests of the two groups. Representatives of the insured membership are interested in maintaining the level of services and benefits. They are not interested in reducing them. On the other hand, business representatives are more critical, but they cannot complain too openly because several years ago they supported legislation to extend coverage and benefits.

Officials' perceptions of what assembly members can do and how they can be influential in the local sickness fund reflect a change in circumstances that was not apparent several decades ago. They recognize that influence flows from formal responsibilities, but they also emphasize the importance of the influence that they can exert over external relations, influence that may be higher than what they can exercise over internal affairs. As members of workers' councils in local institutions or in business management, they can mobilize and inform coworkers and community groups about what the fund does. "This approach is the best guarantee that a social and health policy can be pursued locally, and we intend to influence it," commented one official. For this reason the dissemination of information and the intensification of public-relations efforts are increasingly important in the community, and all funds pursue this strategy of mobilization. There is a clear awareness among officials of the funds, as there is by national and state leaders, that the perception of the general sickness funds (AOK) as the traditional fund of the poor and lower socioeconomic strata continues to be widespread and therefore needs to be changed. As pragmatists, local officials realize that they cannot afford to pursue one strategy directed at only one particular constituency. Because good relations with local providers and hospitals are considered essential in serving the membership of the funds, local officials direct their strategies at several constituencies. Close and good contacts with providers (that is, physicians, dentists, hospitals, and suppliers of medical equipment) are considered as important as access to and good relationships with local government and the local press. Finally, the distribution of information and newsletters to elected board and assembly members as well as to the membership of the fund is an activity in which all local sickness funds are heavily engaged. In light of increasing competition with other funds, open discussions offering plausible explanations of why the general sickness fund has higher contribution rates than its competitor are considered essential aspects of the strategy of mobilization.

What interest do assembly members evince in the affairs of the fund? One criterion used to assess the interests of assembly members in influencing fund affairs and policy involves an examination of the average attendance rate at meetings. But taking the attendance rate as a reflection of the level of interest in and concern for the fund—an approach that is helpful in other situations—is meaningless in this context. To avoid the possibility that surprise votes may occur at meetings, legislation for some time has provided for the election of "A" and "B" representatives, who replace regular members who are unable to attend. Therefore the high attendance rate, which was said to be about 95 percent by some and 100 percent by others, is not surprising. How often regular members are replaced by deputies is not known.

Individual evaluations of the interests of the members of the sickness fund assembly in operations and policymaking ranged widely among officials. Some reported that representatives of business were considerably more interested in fund affairs than were trade union representatives. Others thought that trade union representatives were more concerned about the fund. Still others assessed the relative interests of employers and employees' representatives to be equal. Irrespective of the assessment, it is a likely function of the officials' political leanings and preferences as well as the working relations that exist between them and political forces. Set forth below are some reactions:

> The interest of assembly members is limited to about three active members.
>
> Both the employer and the employee representatives are very interested in decision-making processes and the management of the fund.
>
> There is an increased desire and interest on the part of the representatives of employees to be informed and to discuss with the administration problems that are of concern to the membership. The employers' interest is limited to a two-hour meeting that usually precedes the main meeting of the board.

The items on the agenda of the assembly and the frequency of their meetings to review and authorize or rubber-stamp policies of the governing board are possible indicators of influence. Generally, agenda items are of a routine and a nonroutine nature. Routine items involve reports pertaining to the execution of such official responsibilities as approving and authorizing the budget and amending the statutes or the work provisions. Nonroutine items concern those topics that seem to be of interest at a particular time only. Such matters include relocating the main office or the field offices to improve working conditions for the staff and improve capacities through which services are provided to members of the fund.

Field material documenting how often the assembly and the committees meet and the topics that they discuss is, admittedly, spotty. Depending on its financial means, each fund, in varying degrees of comprehensiveness, reports on a range of issues. Irrespective of comprehensiveness, the reports project a picture of ongoing activities and events considered worth reporting to the public. In this sense, the narrative set forth in the next few pages is a description of items of interest not only to the assembly but to the board and the sickness fund as an organization.

Usually each assembly meets twice a year, once around June and once in December. At the June meeting the assembly approves and votes on closing accounts, and at the December meeting it authorizes the budget for the coming year. Depending on circumstances, which differ greatly from fund to fund, additional meetings may be convened. We also found evidence that many assemblies met only once a year in the past. Causes for holding extraordinary and additional meetings varied. Although most officials think that contribution rates should be calculated once for the calendar year, the finances of several funds, especially in the early 1970s, required additional meetings to approve raises in contributions because revenues did not cover expenditures. The topic of local government reform was on the agenda of the assemblies of several funds. Usually the impact of reform is reflected in a loss or a gain in membership and a corresponding shift in the composition of desirable to less desirable membership groups. Financial and organizational consequences, such as the need to reassign staff members to different divisions, were reported.

Other recurring and attention-getting topics were the frequent changes in federal program stipulations concerning the health-insurance program and the other social-insurance programs that funds administer. Federal programs are directly linked to additional staffing and hiring requirements. Within a two-year period, from 1973 to 1975, the AOK Düsseldorf reported that thirty-two staff members were hired.[8] In its comprehensive report on administration—the only one of its kind available—the fund summarized the effects that changes in federal law and administrative guidelines as well as a new emphasis on client orientation had had on staff developments since 1973. Because the description of direct federal impacts is detailed, it is of more than passing interest. It reveals the direct link between federal activities and local events at the fund level, in particular its relationship to the rehabilitation program passed in 1974.

Changes in the registration provisions for the social-insurance programs and those pertaining to the field auditing of registration required the hiring of five employees. Four experts on awards and two on contributions were hired for the administration of the rehabilitation program. The inclusion of students in the general public health-insurance program resulted in the hiring of one staff member. Dispensing improved services to clients, working longer hours in branch offices, providing technical assistance to wage officers in firms, and improving public relations required four employees. Administering the quality-control on medical appliances required one staff member. The most dramatic impact occurred in the area of data processing and management. An organizational unit for data processing was developed, and ten staff members were hired for it. With a total of eighteen employees, the office on data processing was the fourth most expensive office in terms of total administrative costs in 1976.

The passage of the *Personalvertretungsgesetz* resulted in the hiring of two staff members to assist the Staff Employees' Council (*Personalrat*) and to follow through by formulating administrative requirements that concern the fund in its capacity as employer. Regular meetings of the staff council with the board committee on personnel require considerable administrative activities. Finally, three staff members were hired to perform miscellaneous activities.

The report indicates other instances of additional work load and/or expenses, although no quantitative indicator was given. For example, the training of top- and middle-level managers and employees who work directly with clients resulted in administrative expenditures. The reduction of the work week from forty-two to forty hours in 1974 affected staff time and costs. It also resulted in the granting of additional vacation days in 1975. Other funds reported similar developments.

Reporting the celebration of anniversaries of staff members who have been affiliated with a sickness fund for thirty, forty, or fifty years is a feature of the annual reports. The reporting of these events, which give rise to the payment of a special bonus to the individuals concerned, indicates the importance of a fund as a long-time employer in a community and the need to disseminate this kind of information to the community. Although one might have expected different degrees of pressure to be exerted to inform the membership in a rural setting as opposed to an urban context, we found that urban and rural funds devoted equal attention to this issue. Other items frequently reported are the resignation or the promotion of staff, the total number of staff members, as well as changes in the officers of the assembly and the board.

Committees of the Assembly

There are several committees that the assembly must establish and others that it may set up. The assembly chooses committee members on the basis of equal representation of the two political constituencies. Usually two business and two trade union representatives constitute the auditing committee, the most important control committee of the assembly. It is mandated by law and is responsible for auditing the accounts and releasing board officials and management from assuming responsibility for any liability associated with the accounts of the preceding year. The information contained in the annual report of one sickness fund made it possible to ascertain who was involved, what the procedure consisted of, and how the auditing committee conducted the audit.

In addition to the four elected members, the chairman of the board, the deputy chairman of the board, and the deputy chairman of the assembly took part in the auditing session. Three management officials (the executive director, the official responsible for internal auditing, and the departmental head) were also present. The auditing session lasted for ninety minutes. At the completion of the session, one assembly member was asked to report to the assembly, to ask for its approval of the audit, and to obtain the release from liability. Prior to this session, the auditing committee reportedly had done two spot checks of the accounts and the administrative record compiled during the previous year.

Like the board, the assembly can set up additional committees and delegate certain responsibilities—provided that they are not law-making responsibilities—that require decisions by the full assembly or the full board. Two kinds of committees exist, a recent division of responsibility. Some committees exercise delegated law-making responsibilities in certain areas specifically assigned to them; they can authorize certain actions without having to report back to the assembly. Other committees have advisory functions only; they recommend which actions they believe the assembly or the board ought to take. The assembly and the board may or may not accept the advisory committees' recommendations. Management is usually present at the meetings of the advisory committee; in many instances both the director and his deputy attend.

Except for the auditing committee, which has a fixed number of four persons, the number of committees and their size vary from fund to fund. Large funds tend to have more committees than small funds, a tendency that characterizes both the assembly and the board. Some funds do not distinguish committees of the assembly from those of the board. By law the assembly must set up the following committees:

auditing committee
committee on complaints
committee on the wage-continuation program (which is confined to business representatives and usually has two subcommittees, financing and budgeting, and statutes)

Assembly committees are hardly more active than the assembly itself. By and large, the reports document that they meet between once and twice a year but by no means regularly. Depending on extraordinary circumstances, committees meet more often. For example, the committee on construction is a surprisingly busy committee in most funds and not only during one time period. The audit committee must meet at least once to review the accounts.

Despite scarce information, two funds reported more extensively on the activities of the assembly and its committees. Table 14.2 shows the number of meetings held by the assembly and the assembly committees of the AOK Düsseldorf. With the exception of the committee on complaints, there was recorded a very slight increase in the number of the meetings of the committees and the assembly in the early 1970s compared to ten and twenty years earlier. The increase may be related to the beginning of financial problems for the funds as they occurred in all general sickness funds, and also to the increased impact of new federal pro-

Table 14.2. Number of Meetings, Assembly and Assembly Committees, AOK Düsseldorf

Institution	*1955*	*1965*	*1972*	*1973*	*1974*	*1975*	*1976*
Assembly as a whole	4	3	3	5	5	2	4
Committee on Financing and Budgeting	–	1	2	5	4	1(2)	2
Committee on Statutes	2	1	3	4	3	2(4)	2
Committee on Accounts	1	2	2	2	2	2	2
Committee on Complaints	12	8				6	
Committee on Wage-Continuation Program (full committee)						2	
Subcommittee on Financing and Budgeting						1	
Subcommittee on Statutes						2	

Source: Personal communication on the years 1955, 1965, and 1975. AOK Düsseldorf, *Bericht 1977,* S. 1, for the years 1972 to 1976.

grams on the administration of the fund. But it may also coincide with the fact that new management took office in 1972 and in 1973.

By way of summary, when the activities of the "legislative" bodies of the assembly and the assembly committees are compared with those of the "executive" branch—a comparison that will be presented in the next section—the assembly emerges as the institution that mainly serves debating, symbolic, and ritualistic functions. The assembly also meets the formal and institutional requirements of the concept of self-governance.

The Board and Its Committees

Federal provisions design a strong role for the board in internal affairs in general and in relation to the assembly in particular. Usually the board informs and reports to the assembly about issues and future problems that may face the sickness fund. The board is responsible for the management of the insurance fund and its policy as well as for representing the fund externally. External relations are of no interest here. The following pages complement what has been presented about the assembly with information about the board and its committees. Because meetings are not public, reporting on the entire range of activities undertaken by the board may be more comprehensive than what we describe here.

Like the assembly, the range of agenda items varies from routine to nonroutine items and from fund to fund. Routine items are those that require the board to make formal decisions authorizing internal or external action. Decisions concerning personnel, approving the budget prepared by management, and formulating and approving contracts with medical and nonmedical providers and hospitals concerning rehabilitation centers or similar facilities are recurring items on the agendas prepared for board meetings. Other recurring items are raising contribution rates and analyzing the results of the yearly account-audit spot check performed by the auditing committee, as well as deliberating representational and organizational questions related to self-governance. Changes in legislation, their consequences for the fund, and solutions devised to overcome difficulties are other regular topics of interest.

Depending on the circumstance of a fund, its location, and the time period studied, nonroutine items also come up for the board's consideration and decision making. For example, setting up a branch office and administrative and organization matters that result from mergers of funds–including decisions about how to share or divide assets–appear important at particular times. Whereas public relations efforts were of little concern in previous decades when they were identified as a nonroutine item, today these concerns and preoccupations about becoming a more service- and client-oriented organization are recurring agenda items.

What Criteria Guide the (S)election of Members of the Board and the Committees? Expertise and affiliation with one political constituency–that is, trade union or business–determine candidacy and election of the members to the board and the committees. Depending on the fund involved, other considerations influence that choice. In theory, attempts are made to involve a cross-section of occupational and professional groups in trade union representation and a cross-section of representatives from local trades and business firms. Rural funds, which usually cover larger territories, must be sensitive to the need for regional representation of groups and enterprises or trades in their areas. In practice, such a cross-section of groups, employers, and regions is difficult to achieve, as most officials acknowledged. In regions where religious affiliation continues to exert extraordinary influence in local politics, the need for Catholic and/or Protestant representation must be satisfied.

For the fund in Düsseldorf, we have obtained information on the provenance and age of board members and on the mix of regional industries on the board: One lawyer works for the employer's association in the region, one comes from Daimler-Benz, the automobile manufacturing firm, one represents an old, well-established downtown department store, and one works for auto industry suppliers. The affiliations of the remaining board members on the employers' side are unknown. Four trade union representatives are trade union officials, one represents the Catholic Movement of the Trade Unions (KAB), and one represents the Protestant church. The representative of the latter speaks on behalf of senior citizens. Business representatives are considerably younger than their trade union and religious counterparts. The average age of business representatives is forty-six, whereas that of trade union representatives is fifty-five.

Like information about the assembly and its committees, information about the board and the frequency of board and committee meetings is neither systematic nor comprehensive for all funds. But on the basis of published reports and field work, one conclusion can be drawn: the board and board committees are the active decision makers in all funds. For example, the assembly of the AOK München met 12 times in a five-year period. During the same period the board met 112 times and covered a total of 1074 agenda items.[9] Table 14.3, a comparison of agenda items and meetings of the board with those of the assembly of the AOK Amberg, confirms this conclusion. The 1955 report characterizes agenda items as provider contracts, personnel, and administration. The 1965 and 1975 reports do not indicate the nature of topics.

Board members are elected to the committees on the basis of parity between business and trade union representatives and in conformity with criteria of competence that governed their election to the board. Because individual funds determine the total number of committees, the number varies from fund to fund and ranges from a minimum of six to a maximum of about ten. Size, special circumstances (such as strong competition emanating from another health-insurance carrier and the corresponding need to improve public relations), and mandated activities and programs seem to determine the total number of committees. Because auditing the accounts and revising the wage-continuation program are prescribed by law, every board maintains two standing committees to discharge those responsibilities. The most regular and recurring board committees are the following:

Contracts with Providers
Personnel
Statutes
Financing and Budgeting

Table 14.3. A Comparison of the Meetings of the Board and the Assembly of the AOK Amberg, 1955–1975

	1955		*1960*		*1965*		*1975*	
	Board	*Assembly*	*Board*	*Assembly*	*Board*	*Assembly*	*Board*	*Assembly*
Frequency of meetings	14	1	9	1	6	2	9	3
Number of agenda items	174	15	n.a.	n.a.	121	16	126	18

Source: Data for 1955, 1965, and 1975 from the fund's annual reports. Data for 1960 from an informal source, 1960.
n.a. = not available.

Construction and Facilities
Auditing
Wage-Continuation Program

In addition, some funds maintain committees on administration and on relations with the press, whereas in others these functions may be taken care of by an organizational division of a fund. Lines of responsibility between a board committee and this organizational division seem to fluctuate.

Apart from the auditing committee and the committee on the wage-continuation program, which must meet, the other committees meet when need and interest are involved. The committees on personnel, contracts, and construction seem to be more active than the others.

Several funds have merged legislative and executive decision-making authority into one committee, although the law provides for their separation. The committee on construction has advisory functions only. Because of the need for frequent and informed meetings between specialists, however, the committee includes members of the assembly and of the board. This committee is usually given authority to commit the financial resources of the fund to construction projects and to major repairs. Formally, the executive director or his deputy or sometimes both serve in advisory capacities. Informally, however, they are the most important participants because they are knowledgeable about the resources of the funds, and they advise accordingly.

The usual number of committee members is four (two from each constituency). Some board committees seem to have more than four members, whereas others seem to have fewer members, that is, one from each constituency only. Field research on one fund identified the members of committees. Of sixteen members who were identified as regular members of the four major committees (statutes, auditing, construction, personnel), three served as regular members on more than one committee. One person served as a regular member on three committees and as a replacement on another. An examination of the names of the replacements showed that only two out of eight were new members: all the remaining replacements were people who served as substitutes on committees of which they were not regular members. The materials on other sickness funds are less extensive, but on the whole, the incidence of overlapping membership, which enables a few members to control activities, may be the norm rather than the exception.

Information on the AOK Düsseldorf provides some interesting insights into committee activities. In 1977 a total of nine regular committees and two subcommittees assisted the full board in discharging its responsibilities. Table 14.4 lists the committees in existence during the

1955–1975 period and identifies the number of meetings of the board and its committees. In the early period of the 1950s the full board appeared to be more active than it was twenty years later. The total number of board committee meetings slowly but steadily increased, from twenty-eight in 1955 to thirty-four in 1976. An unusually busy time characterized the period between 1973 and 1975.

Table 14.4. Number of Meetings of the Board and Its Committees

	1955	*1965*	*1972*	*1973*	*1974*	*1975*	*1976*	*1978*
Board	15	12	12	18	13	9	11	18
Board committees								
Personnel	11	11	12	17	5	8	4	
Construction	1	11	3	5	7	7	7	
Financing and Budgeting	3	2	5	9	10	5	7	
Statutes	2	–	5	5	5	2	6	
Data Processing	–	–	–	–	–	3	2	
Auditing			3	4	2	2	2	
Representation on the Board of the VdO			2	2	2	2	2	
Board Committee on the Wage-Continuation Program							2	
Subcommittee on Financing and Budgeting							2	
Subcommittee on Statutes							1	

Source: Personal communication for the years 1955, 1965, and 1975

The data seem to suggest that shifts in the location of responsibilities and work load from the full board to the committees might have taken place. But the full board met eighteen times in 1978, which amounted to about twice a month, allowing for the vacation periods of Christmas and Easter. The busy period from 1973 to 1975 coincided with a change in management and with extraordinary circumstances such as rising expenditures. The contribution rate was increased three times within an eighteen-month period, from 8.8 to 9.5 percent in July 1973, to 9.9 percent in February 1974, and to 11.7 percent in January 1975. Because raises in contribution rates require the assembly's approval, the assembly met more often during that period. At the same time benefits, particularly dental care and rehabilitation (including diagnostic, therapeutic, and rehabilitative care), were also increased.

Management

When the subject of the authority of management vis-à-vis the assembly and the board is approached, parallels come to mind—for example, the widely analyzed situation involving designated and actual decision makers in public policy formation and implementation, and the increasingly important role of the bureaucracy in both (although often we do not know the boundaries of this role). Despite the low profile accorded to management in the law and in the statutes, it is apparent from the previous sections of this chapter that top management plays a crucial role in a local sickness fund. Of course, the law places numerous constraints on management: a myriad of program stipulations, employment contracts, and provider contracts circumscribes the scope of decision making. The top members of management are considered permanent staff and represent continuity and institutional stability. They also represent expertise because they have detailed knowledge and information. The roles that executive directors play determine the affairs of sickness funds and provide a clue to the presence or the absence of conflict. Obviously, an evaluation of self-governance in sickness funds that excluded the role of management vis-à-vis the political decision makers who are also constrained by federal and state provisions would be two-dimensional because it would prevent the analyst from gaining insight into the significance of self-governance in practice as well as in theory.

Formally and in social-science literature (except that written for trainees and practioners), top management and the internal administration of a sickness fund hardly exist.[10] The law simply states that "the executive director is responsible full time for the administration." Court rulings have delineated management's areas of responsibilities:[11]

1. to serve as intermediary between providers of services and fund members and to make certain that health services are available to the membership;
2. to secure the necessary financial resources to pay for services received by patients/members.

What does top management, that is, the executive director, actually do in the context of providing services and collecting contributions? Indeed, collecting contributions is one important activity of the staff of a fund. The other is the payment of bills for services received by the members.

Contributions to the public health-insurance program constitute on a national average about 95 percent of the total revenues of a fund. Payments for all services absorb a similar percentage of total revenues.[12] Because of the complex, interrelated operational aspects involved in day-to-day management with respect to these two functions, we cannot provide a definitive answer in the context of this chapter. But we will begin by examining the major responsibilities of the executive director.

In training courses, students learn that the executive director is responsible for the general administration of the fund and its branch offices. He acquires and makes available the financial, organizational, and related resources necessary for that purpose. He manages the fund's properties and the facilities. He is responsible for balancing the budget and for taking whatever steps are necessary to ensure that revenues cover expenditures in line with legal and statutory provisions and decisions made by the board and the assembly. In other words, he is responsible for the fund's budget and for the accounts. If members, suppliers, or providers violate the law or the statutes, he must suggest to the board that fines and penalties, including the filing of official charges, be imposed. One of top management's most important concerns is hiring and promoting staff members and, in extreme cases, giving notice to fund employees. But, in the formal discharge of his responsibilities, he cannot act alone. The executive director must secure the signature of the chairman of the board.

Because contribution rates are calculated on the basis of the basic wage, and this in turn is based on the actual wage, the director must formally determine basic and actual wages. That determination is important in calculating contributions not only to the public health-insurance program but also to other social-insurance programs such as retirement, unemployment, and accident. Except for the fact that employers and employees each pay half the amount of the contribution, national provisions on income ceilings and maximum contribution rates for these social and health-insurance programs differ.

If a health-insurance fund yields responsibility for a member of the fund because the member has changed his address or because funds were merged and now cater to a different geographic constituency, the director must serve notice to that effect. He must refer the former member to the appropriate fund.

He must negotiate agreements with businesses specifying how and where they must register employees for the various social-security programs administered by the fund. If firms are late in paying contributions to these programs, top management can authorize and set new deadlines. Top management is authorized to waive fines for different kinds of violations and can impose change and cancel default fees. Finally, top management can authorize or reject sick-pay allowances in case of ineligibility.

Trainees in a general sickness fund soon learn that the executive director assumes a variety of additional responsibilities that students may not learn about in correspondence courses or in seminars.[13] As top manager, not only does he serve in legal and administrative capacities—that is, nonpolitical functions that the law and German terminology portray him as performing—but he also serves in a fundamentally political capacity by engaging in both internal and external relations with trade unions, employers' associations, organized medicine, public agencies, other social-insurance carriers, and, finally, the local media. There was a consensus among interviewed officials that compared to ten or fifteen years ago, the executive director today usually spends a higher portion of his time on external relations than on internal relations. Accordingly, responsibilities for internal affairs are shifting to the deputy director and other members of the management staff.

One prime responsibility of the executive director is projecting for the board and the assembly the likely consequences of any decision they might take, for example, with respect to the budget, the membership, or the contribution rates. To perform this service, management must acquire information about national legislative and regulatory developments in the fields of health and social policy, collective-bargaining agreements, and provider contracts, which involves the expenditure of a great deal of time. At the same time, management must pay attention to local developments and changes in membership and morbidity. If there is agreement that giving advice and disseminating information to the membership, the board, and to the assembly, as well as setting the agenda of board and assembly meetings are exercises of influence, then top management and the administration are influential decision makers vis-à-vis the political leadership, although, by law and by statutes, the responsibilities of the board and the assembly are comprehensive and leave little room for autonomous decision making by the administration.

Officials in one fund reported spending about one week per month working for the board. This includes preparing for board meetings and implementing its decisions. For each meeting day, officials estimated allocating about two full days, excluding time spent by other staff members. Preparation requires more time and attention than implementing decisions of the board, but the implementation of board decisions may be as time consuming as preparing for decisions. If the board decides, for example, that the committee on construction or the committee on contracts with providers ought to look into an issue before it comes up for a decision, management faces a work load similar to what would be involved if it were preparing for full board meetings.

The executive director attends board meetings as a nonvoting member. He works more closely with and through board members than with members of the assembly. But as a rule, board members discuss with the chairman and the deputy chairman of the assembly items on the agenda prior to the meetings of the assembly in an effort to reconcile potential conflicts. The existence of two political constituencies on the board and the assembly makes a difference for fund managers. They do not always prevail over one or the other or even both institutions.

Although the federal provisions and the statutes are fairly clear about the responsibilities of the director and those of the board, some of their responsibilities overlap. How are these responsibilities divided, and who resolves conflicts, if they arise? Reactions to this question ranged from a repetition of formalistic and legalistic statements about the allocation of responsibilities, which the previous sections on formal responsibilities identified, to some tentative assessments of what the relationship between management and the board of a sickness fund was in the past and is likely to be in the future. Following are some paraphrased responses:

> Responsibilities between the board and the administration are delineated clearly. Relations between the board and the administration are very good, in part because of the expertise of the executive director and the trust of the board in this expertise.
>
> The statutes outline the areas of responsibility of the board and the executive director. Usually one sticks to it. The board is not interested in interfering with routine administration. Promotion of the staff is a responsibility of the board. In the past there were no jurisdictional conflicts.
>
> It is difficult to draw a clear-cut dividing line between the board and the administration. Up to the present the fund had ten to twelve board meetings a year. Contracts were sanctioned and staff was promoted on the recommendation of and information provided by the executive director. This position is likely to change in the future. There are tendencies to limit the autonomy of the executive director by imposing restrictions on him, by having a more activist board, and by putting management in a straitjacket.
>
> With an average of four to six hours of work by the board every month, it is easy to understand that management must take the initiative regarding daily routine work and representation in the community. We need to be active outside the organization of the sickness fund. To achieve this, we need political representatives who are willing to fight externally, for example, in the context of daily hospital charges.

Some statutes of sickness funds define restrictively and others more flexibly the roles of the executive director vis-à-vis the board. However, specificity or flexibility in the allocation of responsibilities hardly matters in day-to-day operations provided no major political conflict exists between the executive director and the board. If it does, statutory provisions gain the importance they have in the decision-making processes of other institutions such as universities. The professional expertise of top management and the staff remains a requirement for and a precondition of effective management, especially in light of the ever-increasing complexity of federal and state program stipulations and court rulings that affect administration. Respect for and appreciation of professional expertise by the members of the board seem to be others. However, the importance of the personalities of the members of the board, irrespective of political orientation, was singled out as the most important difference in management's interactions with the board and the assembly.

In the perception of one official, frictions between management and the board do not exist. He described the relationship between management and the majority of relatively young and modern-minded board members as being good and cooperative. The administrative leadership style centers on regularly informing the board about all current issues and discussing openly the ramifications because, in his opinion, an open leadership style has two important consequences: "Everything runs more smoothly for the administration. And the political decision makers are not suspicious of management." He seemed to believe that management got the necessary support and attributed the absence of conflict between management and the board largely to open communications and discussions.

Recent legislation politicized the position of the executive director by mandating his election by the assembly, an enactment that superseded the requirement that he be appointed by the board. In addition, attempts are under way to activate self-governance in all social-insurance carriers, that is, in the respective national, state, and local organizations. Evaluations by officials concerning whether these developments might make a difference for administrative leadership differed widely. Because board members prefer the status quo, nothing will change, opined on official. Another official commented that all parties involved needed to play more political games, especially with respect to the (s)election of an executive director and the political moves that he might have to make after his election vis-à-vis members of the board and the assembly. The right to nominate candidates for the position of director remains with the board. Active board members will have to bargain with the assembly chairman or his deputy to secure the assembly's support for the candidate of the board's choice. Provided one behaves politically, there is no insurmountable barrier, was another opinion. These explanations are plausible because the dividing lines on policy issues and financial and administrative matters set apart representatives of employers from those of trade unions rather than the board from the assembly, and these dividing lines have always existed. Because of the importance of these two political constituencies, it is reasonable to assume that directors have always been important political players in the context of a sickness fund, especially ten or twenty years ago, when local sickness funds were able to decide benefits and policy issues that were more important than they are today.

In the past, directors usually were given unlimited informal authority on personnel matters, on implementing the health regulations, and in relation to business and other employers. The possibility that this authority and the right to propose staff members for promotion on the basis of merit may be lost was one concern expressed. Another concern related to whether sickness funds will be able to continue the practice of recruiting committed and professionally competent directors or be impelled in the future to acquiesce in selecting only politically motivated ones.

Regarding social elections, the executive director is supposed to keep a low profile and to remain neutral between the two political camps. He has no formal authority to propose candidates or to influence elections. But it would be unrealistic to expect him to be indifferent about who is elected to the self-governing bodies, especially to the board. Much of what he does requires the board's support. Members of the board can be strong supporters, and they can also be obstructors, delayers, and troublemakers. In a way, an executive director's effectiveness and strength depend on his relationship with the board. For this reason, management cannot afford not to be interested in who is elected and placed on the board. With whom they informally discuss candidates depends, of course, on the political support that a director may give to business or trade unions in national, state, and local politics. Because of the politics practiced in the sickness fund, and in light of the fact that executive directors have to work with members of both groups, their informal contacts are likely to extend to both sides. Whether one reported initiative is called good sense, willingness to cooperate, or simply cooptation is of no significance. The initiative reveals political pragmatism. Because of competition from another fund in the district served by the general sickness fund, lobbying efforts directed at some apparently receptive members of the board and the assembly finally succeeded in securing the candidacy and placement of a member of that competitor on the list for (s)election.

The process of approving candidates on one list and thus of securing their (s)election by the two corporate groups in the funds prior to the election was given as one important explanation of why members exhibit low interest in fund affairs in general and little interest at all in elections in particular. Political leaders and other interested political groups recognize the cause and the effect of low interest on the part of people in the affairs of sickness funds and other social-insurance carriers. They intend to change this, and, for this reason, innovations in the governance of funds seem likely. But we had a revealing response on the part of one official who commented, "This system worked well. Good heavens, I am glad we had it. Social elections cost a lot of money, and what are they to achieve?" Is he simply an old timer and supporter of the status quo? Or did he as local implementer point to crucial considerations? The answer to both questions may be yes.

CONCLUDING COMMENTS

This section serves two purposes: It summarizes important conclusions and indicates the likely development of sickness funds in light of these conclusions. The summary reiterates only what bears on this development.

This chapter took a close look at the major decision makers in a general sickness fund, the division of responsibilities between them, and the actual exercise of these responsibilities in decision making and in controlling the financial and organizational resources of a general sickness fund. Field evidence on the same operational aspects of fund governance reinforces the general conclusions in some literature on social- and health-insurance carriers. Indeed, the materials add more support to the argument that a deep chasm exists between the claims for Selbstverwaltung and its realization in the day-to-day operations of sickness funds.

Decision makers encounter numerous and insurmountable obstacles to autonomous decision making and priority setting that are imposed directly and indirectly by the widening scope and complexity of federal program stipulations, state provisions, and court rulings. Local decisions and local actions are constrained by provisions on health and social policy, conditions of employment, and compensation of staff, as well as by state contracts relating to provider reimbursement, medical supplies, and related services.

In summary, the autonomy exercised by sickness funds in determining services and benefits, in controlling their manpower resources, and in allocating resources on the basis of particular priorities has slowly but steadily been taken away. Decisions about services and benefits, which absorb about 95 percent of a fund's revenues, are made by external actors. Although the financing and the administration of the health-insurance program remain the province of sickness funds (contributions are the only source of revenue, unlike the situation with respect to the other social-insurance programs), sickness funds exercise no real judgment in setting contributions independent of the amount needed to pay for the bundle of services set by federal and state decision makers and to cover the costs of these services, which are determined by providers. Funds must set contributions as high as necessary to balance their budgets.

The pressures to which sickness funds have been exposed lately can be considered to be of three kinds. Federal legislators and regulators and state supervisory authorities are increasingly deciding who should be members of sickness funds, what funds are to do, and how they are to conduct business. Externally negotiated contracts have determined the price that sickness funds have to pay for the services that their members receive. Finally, because they are an integral part of local communities, sickness funds are increasingly exposed to local challenges and pressures. Evidence from the field suggests that in responding to them, sickness funds attempt to do all three things. They report on the increasing financial and administrative burdens that result from external decisions and agreements, with which they have to abide. They raise and grant additional benefits in areas over which they continue to exercise some degree of control, such as transportation allowances, dental subsidies, and preventive measures. Finally, they all engage in local health-related activities, such as organizing health exhibitions and lectures and discussions.

With respect to individual components of the governance structure, the infrequent meetings of the assembly are hardly conducive to making it an important decision maker, although it has a few responsibilities—such as the authority to approve the statutes, the work provisions, and the budget—that it exercises on the advice of and at the direction of the board and management. As a "legislative" institution, the assembly serves symbolic and ritualistic functions, but its members are important political brokers in relation to their coworkers, employers, and related social and political groups in the community.

National decision makers and citizens seem to get from general sickness funds whatever the board and management decide rather than what the assembly thinks appropriate in dealing with increasing restrictions, cutting through red tape, and avoiding paralysis. How management prepares information and what kinds of information it prepares in proposing alternative strategies seem to influence board decisions and actions. In turn, the way in which information is received and processed by individual board members influences the operations in which directors can engage. Expertise and political skills in dealing with influential board members seem to be responsible for holding the system together. Future developments undoubtedly will affect the position of management, enhancing or decreasing the administration's capability to act effectively.

To recapitulate three developments that are likely to be the source of future developments: (1) the gradual erosion and abolition of independent authority and control over financial, organizational, and manpower resources; (2) the strengthening of Selbstverwaltung through the election of executive directors by the assembly, in lieu of simple appointment by the board, and other mobilization strategies; and (3) increased competition from other insurance carriers and the corresponding need to enhance visibility in the community by developing a better public-relations image through organizing "tooth fairy" programs and related health-education programs.

National decision makers intended to strengthen the capacity of funds in order to achieve organizational effectiveness and to influence the distribution and the availability of services. Although not all aspects that bear on the capacities of the sickness funds were examined in this chapter, this much seems clear. If funds are to respond to community pressures and competition from other sickness funds and influence the delivery and the distribution of health services to their members, they need more authority and discretion than they now have. On the other hand, local sickness funds are likely to be exposed to additional national pressures. If the idea of strengthening Selbstverwaltung gains adherents, support may well be mobilized in the national and state-level associations as well as in the local sickness funds. Judging by past political developments, national and state political forces have been successful over local forces in imposing their preferences. If this process is repeated, local sickness funds will be less capable of developing what some national circles consider to be the right response to local pressures.

NOTES

1. Florian Tennstedt, *Soziale Selbstverwaltung,* Band 2 (Bonn: Verlag der Ortskrankenkassen, 1977), pp. 49–50. See also Christian von Ferber, "Soziale Selbstverwaltung–Fiktion oder Chance?" and Harald Bogs, "Strukturprobleme der Selbstverwaltung einer modernen Sozialversicherung" in Harald Bogs and Christian von Ferber, *Soziale Selbstverwaltung,* Band 1 (Bonn: Verlag der Ortskrankenkassen, 1977).
2. Hans Töns, *Grundausbildung für den Krankenkassendienst* (Sankt Augustin: Asgard Verlag), 12. überarbeitete Auflage, Juli 1980.
3. Viertes Buch der Sozialgesetzgebung–Gemeinsame Vorschriften für die Sozialversicherung (SGB-IV).
4. Wirtschafts- und Sozialwissenschaftliches Institut des Deutschen Gewerkschaftsbundes, *Sozialpolitik und Selbstverwaltung* (Köln: Bund-Verlag, 1977).
5. Allgemeine Ortskrankenkasse München, *Satzung.*
6. Bundesverband der Ortskrankenkassen et al., *Aufbau und Organisation der Sozialversicherung,* August 1978; and *Soziale Krankenversicherung,* 8/1979, 10/1979, and 5/1980.

7. Bundesverband der Ortskrankenkassen, *Die Ortskrankenkassen 1975,* pp. 128–129.
8. Allgemeine Ortskrankenkasse Düsseldorf, *Bericht über die Untersuchung der Verwaltungskosten der AOK Düsseldorf,* Januar 1977, pp. 82–83.
9. Allgemeine Ortskrankenkasse München, *Geschäftsbericht 1967–1971.*
10. See references in notes 1 and 4.
11. *Soziale Krankenversicherung,* 8/1979, p. 310.
12. Bundesverband der Ortskrankenkassen, *Die Ortskrankenkassen 1975.*
13. *Soziale Krankenversicherung,* 8/1979: pp. 307–310.

REFERENCES

Allgemeine Ortskrankenkasse Amberg. *Geschäftsbericht 1975.*

———. *Geschäftsbericht 1965.*

———. *Geschäfts-und Rechnungsergebnisse 1955.*

———. *Satzung der AOK Amberg.*

Allgemeine Ortskrankenkasse Brilon in Olsberg. *Geschäftsberichte* für die Jahre 1972–1977.

Allgemeine Ortskrankenkasse Düsseldorf. *Bericht über die Untersuchung der Verwaltungskosten der AOK Düsseldorf,* Januar 1977.

———. *Bericht über die Untersuchung der Verwaltungskosten des Jahres 1976.*

———. *Satzung der AOK Düsseldorf.*

Allgemeine Ortskrankenkasse Hochsauerlandkreiss. *Haushaltsplan für das Haushaltsjahr 1979.*

Allgemeine Ortskrankenkasse Siegerland-Wittgenstein. *Das Geschäftsjahr 1977.*

———. *Das Geschäftsjahr 1976.*

———. *Satzung der AOK Siegerland-Wittgenstein.*

Allgemeine Ortskrankenkasse München. *Statistischer Bericht für das Jahr 1977.*

———. *Geschäftsbericht 1967–1971.*

———. *Geschäftsbericht 1957–1966.*

———. *Organisationsplan.*

———. *Satzung. Stand 1. Januar 1978.*

Allgemeine Ortskrankenkasse Weiden i.d. OPf. *Haushaltsplan mit Erläuterungen für das Geschäftsjahr 1979.*

———. *Geschäftsbericht 1977.*

———. *Satzung.*

PART IV

Conclusion

In light of the contributions to this volume, Rudolf Klein proposes a research agenda for the systematic study of comparative health-policy research. He suggests two specific areas for cross-national research about which little is known: the diffusion of technological innovations and organizational experiments in response to them. Fundamental to his analytical framework is a distinction that Klein draws between medical care—the delivery of high-cost and manpower-intensive technical services—and health care—the provision of mainly social support. Both are embedded in a different set of factors. In Klein's view, most cases in this volume indicate that medical technologies are primarily international in character, but they do create demands for organizational innovations domestically. Despite a convergence of problems, he sees no convergence of solutions across nations. He urges, therefore, that research identify those factors that determine organizational strategies that individual countries have adopted in attempts to deal with these pressures. According to him, we need to know more about the positive and negative incentives used to bring about organizational innovations. As a first step in explaining the differential capacities of central governments to control the diffusion of technological innovations, Klein proposes a typology that analyzes the relationship between control capabilities and the political, social, and institutional characteristics of particular countries.

Chapter 15

Prospects and Problems in the Comparative Study of Health-Services Innovation

Rudolf Klein

INTRODUCTION

How can countries systematically learn from one another's experience in the field of health policy? Is it possible to move beyond national case studies that may be useful in provoking thought or in stimulating imitation but from which it is difficult to derive conclusions of general applicability? This paper represents a first, tentative attempt to address these questions or, to be more precise, to discuss an analytical framework for such an exercise and the scope for crossnational research in light of the various papers presented in this volume.

Health services are ideal candidates for crossnational studies of innovation. The technology (in the widest, most comprehensive sense of that term) of medical care is international: There is a shared body of knowledge, agreed ways of doing things, the free movement of ideas, and a considerable degree of professional mobility. No country can isolate itself from what is happening elsewhere. On the one hand, innovations in the practice of medical care developed in one country are likely to diffuse across national frontiers. On the other hand, many such innovations—particularly in the field of drugs and technological hardware—are produced by multinational companies using international marketing strategies.

In these respects, health services are unique among social services. However, it is important to draw a crucial distinction. Health services have two components that, although interwoven in practice, should be distinguished analytically. The first is the element of *medical* care, that is, the delivery of a technical service involving the application of specific procedures to particular conditions. The second is the element of *health* care: The provision of support—largely social in character—in those cases in which medical care may do little more than prolong life.

We come to the peculiar paradox presented by the health services, which are distinguished by a process of continuous, spontaneous innovation in the field of techniques that transcends national boundaries—a process, as T. R. Marmor suggests in his paper, deeply rooted in the ideology of the medical profession. The problem appears to be not so much how to encourage innovation but how to control it. Technical innovation creates social problems, notably, by prolonging the lives of those who require some form of social support, posing the problem of how to stimulate innovation in the social organization of health care. Technical innovation thus creates a demand for organizational innovation both to control its use and to cope with its consequences. Whereas technical innovation is primarily international in character, organizational innovation is likely to be shaped by social, political, and institutional factors peculiar to individual countries.

It is important to stress the convergence of problems faced by health services in all advanced industrial nations. There are shared economic constraints. On the one hand, the slowing down of economic growth has imposed sharp limits on public expenditure nearly everywhere (1). On the other hand, irrespective of increases in scale or scope, the health services—like all manpower-intensive public services—will continue to absorb a larger portion of national income because of the fact that conventional national accounting makes no allowance for increasing productivity to be set off against rising wages and salaries (2). Consequently, it is not surprising that there is a general preoccupation with cost containment (3). There are shared demographic factors. Almost everywhere the growth in the number of elderly people is generating pressures on health services. There are shared political factors: The demand for equality of access to health services, as several commentators suggest, may make it difficult to limit the availability of and the expenditures for new technologies.

To underline the convergence of problems is not to suggest a convergence of solutions or that a comparative study of innovations will lead to the adoption of the same strategies. On the contrary, because so many exogenous conditions are shared, it is particularly interesting to study the endogenous system variables: the way in which different countries handle the same problems. Some of these innovative strategies may be system specific, that is, so deeply embedded in the organizational structure of a particular health system that they are not exportable. Other strategies may be system independent, that is, detachable because they are self-contained and not contingent on a variety of other factors that may prove difficult to manipulate. The challenge for policy-oriented researchers is to analyze innovative strategies in the context of the limitations imposed by the national political and cultural environments in which specific systems function.

CONTROLLING TECHNOLOGICAL INNOVATION

We lack an accurate and a precise vocabulary for discussing technological innovation. To rephrase the problem, we have no accepted taxonomy of technological innovation, and the development of such a system of classification should be given high priority on any research agenda. Consequently, any discussion is likely to blur the various meanings of technology (4) when the work is applied to the field of medical care. For example, the term can be used to describe clinical techniques, that is, the strategies pursued by clinicians in treating patients. In this sense, day surgery could be described as a technological innovation (and one, moreover, that tends to diminish rather than increase pressures on resources). Technology may be used to describe surgical procedures: coronary bypass surgery is frequently cited. Another instance would be hip-replacement surgery. Technology is used most frequently to describe hardware such as the CAT scanner, although it is important to emphasize that the magnitude of the cost of individual items of equipment may be a poor guide to the importance of a particular technological innovation. Consider, for instance, the heart pacemaker, the cost of which is small but the economic implications (both positive and negative) of its availability are considerable.

The sheer diversity of the technological changes that are taking place suggests that a variety of organizational responses may be required. It is important to emphasize the difference between those innovations that are capital intensive because they require the purchase of expensive equipment and those that may generate extra demands on resources through the cumulative effect of small-scale decisions made by individual clinicians. In the former case, those health systems that exercise close central control over capital expenditure appear to offer the most interesting model. Thus both Britain and France seem to have been successful in limiting the diffusion of CAT scanners because the center is able to ration the allocation of capital. In the second case, however, there is much less clear-cut evidence about which system, if any, is best designed to influence clinical innovation. The crucial question appears to be the nature of incentives that are built into various health systems and the extent to which they are manipulable.

Thus in the case of the British NHS, which requires doctors to work within fixed budgets primarily for salaries rather than fees, there are no direct financial incentives to encourage the precipitate adoption of technological innovations (although there may be professional incentives if the adoption of methods or techniques enhances prestige and reputation). But in the case of systems based on the payment of fees for services rendered, such as that of the United States, the balance of incentives appears to work in the opposite direction. Technological innovation—in particular, the adoption of procedures—may be a way of swelling medical incomes. Moreover, the same point can be made about institutional behavior. In the case of Britain, individual hospitals have no incentive to advertise the availability of special facilities: The structure of their incentives encourages them to minimize, not maximize, their work loads (because their budgets will not increase if they attract more patients). In contrast, American hospitals operate in a competitive market and have every incentive to attract new patients by publicizing the availability of new technologies. The system of incentives may help to explain the failure of attempts to exercise control in the United States by regulating capital investment: There is an imbalance between the machinery of regulation and the structure of incentives.

It is important to distinguish between negative and positive incentives, between the ability of those responsible for health systems to discourage the premature adoption of technological innovations and their success in encouraging the diffusion of innovations once their effectiveness and efficiency have been demonstrated. Thus although the British NHS is strong in generating negative incentives, it is weak in generating positive incentives. Central policymakers lack the means—apart from exhortation—of promoting the diffusion of innovations that are judged to be desirable, for example, day surgery. In contrast, systems based on the payment of fees appear to offer more direct opportunities for influencing clinical practice. By changing the rewards for particular procedures, it should be possible to influence the pattern of medical practice. But it is far from evident that this change happens in practice (5), and more studies are needed in order to investigate the extent to which different systems have the capacity to manipulate their fee schedules to discourage untested innovations and to encourage desired innovations. What evidence there is seems to suggest that most fee schedules tend to have built-in biases toward encouraging the uncritical use of technology.

This point implies a decisive limitation on the adaptive capacity of health systems: the attitude of the medical profession and its political power. If fee schedules reflect the priorities of the medical profession and if these schedules are biased toward the technological imperative, then it may be very difficult to change them without waging the kind of head-on battle that governments everywhere will be eager to avoid because they cannot, as past evidence suggests (6), be certain of winning. Moreover the value system and the structure of prestige of the medical profession are crucial even in those systems that do not operate on a fee-for-service basis. If the British NHS has found it very difficult, as R. G. S. Brown argued in his paper, to change the balance of allocating resources among different client groups in favor of the elderly and the chronically disadvantaged, one reason is that the balance of power within the medical profession tends to favor the traditional, technology-intensive sectors of acute care.

Any comparative study of strategies for coping with technological innovation must rest on an analysis of health services as political systems. Their adaptive capacity depends largely on the balance of power that exists among a variety of different interests, among whom the medical profession is only one, for, to pursue the example quoted above, the seeming ability of doctors everywhere to defend a system biased toward the technological imperative depends less on the "power" of the medical profession (seen in isolation) than on its ability to build a coalition for such a policy. On the one hand, there is the interest of the health-service unions in defending the existing patterns of distributing jobs. On the other hand, there is the widespread evidence of public support for the rapid diffusion of technological innovation, irrespective of evaluation. Even in the case of the British NHS, the official policy of restricting the introduction of CAT scanners has been partly negated by public generosity in presenting the health service with free machines (7). In other words, there appears to be an imbalance between the constituencies for rapid innovation and the constituencies for systematic evaluation and controlled diffusion. Again, only researchers engaged in crossnational studies can investigate the relative strengths of these constituencies in different health systems operating in different political environments.

Political factors seem to impose limitations on the scope for institutional innovation. The road to control runs through evaluation—a complex and difficult process, as David Banta's paper shows. Unquestionably, there is a need for comparative studies of how different health systems cope with the problem of evaluation, in particular, the policies and roles of research councils and of central departments. Similarly, there appears to be a case for investigating the opportunities that may exist for the international dissemination of evaluation: If technological innovation is international, could not technological evaluation be made so? But improving the institutional bases of evaluation may produce only a limited impact if political and professional pressures for rapid diffusion pull in the opposite direction. Therefore, the problem of controlling technological innovation seems to be less a quesion of inventing institutions or introducing organizational checks—necessary though these devices may be—than of creating the kind of political coalition that would generate countervailing pressures against the present constellation of health-service interests.

The other reason for stressing the importance of analyzing how to control technological innovation through political processes is that the decisions involved cannot be determined solely on the bases of studies of the clinical efficacy or cost-effectiveness of using particular machinery, procedures, or techniques. Must all life-saving or life-enhancing techniques be generally available? Different countries seem to be giving different answers, witness the variations in the availability of renal dialysis (8), about which Britain, for example, has taken a deliberate decision to restrict access. If, in turn, access is restricted—whether as an act of deliberate policy to save resources or because of shortages of skilled technicians—who is to determine the criteria: the professional service providers at the periphery or the central policymakers? And what, in turn, should those criteria be? To make these points is to suggest that any comparative analysis of technological innovations must be anchored in knowledge of the societal values of the countries concerned and the political structure that determines who shall articulate those values.

EXPERIMENTS IN ORGANIZATIONAL INNOVATION

The convergence in the problems faced by health services everywhere, which was noted at the beginning of this paper, is leading to a convergence in the organizational strategies adopted to meet at least one important aspect of the problem. It is not merely technological innovations that raise the issue of how to ration scarce resources, although they have certainly added to the pressures that have put this issue on the agenda, it is the distributional aspect of who gets what medical or health care. The search for organizational strategies designed to bring about an acceptable distribution of resources reflects not only the awareness that demand will always exceed supply, and that therefore explicit rationing criteria are required, but that political pressures are increasing for equal access to health care.

There are three main dimensions to the distribution of health-service resources. First is the geographical distribution of resources. Second is the distribution among specific groups of beneficiaries (e.g., the mentally ill or the elderly). Finally, there is the distribution of facilities, or of access to any supply of health resources (i.e., differences in the availability of facilities).

Organizational strategies have been mainly concerned with the geographical distribution of resources. One of the main attempts at policy innovation over the past decade has been the effort to devise formulas according to which resources are distributed geographically on the basis of what are perceived to be equitable criteria. Almost all health services in advanced industrial societies have experimented with criteria related to manpower, numbers of beds and equipment that have been designed to improve the geographical distribution of resources.

These experiments seem to offer considerable scope both for comparative studies and for cross-national learning. In particular, there seems to be an opportunity for countries to learn from one another's mistakes. For example, Jean de Kervasdoué's paper criticizes the current French policy of mandating norms for equipment, the number of doctors, and bed capacity. As he rightly argues, these requirements assume that a given package of resources will necessarily produce the same output of health care, whereas the determining factor is the way in which those resources are used by service providers. British experience seems to be relevant. Britain started experimenting with norms in the early 1960s but has since moved toward a more flexible system designed to bring about equity in the allocation of financial resources to different parts of the country without attempting to prescribe in detail how these resources will be used (9). Indeed, given the possibility that some resources can be substituted for others (e.g., doctors and nurses and beds earmarked for the elderly and acute general beds that may be occupied largely by the elderly), there is a great deal to be said for such an approach.

However, whether the preferred solution is a policy of rigid norms tied to specific kinds of provision or a strategy of equity in allocating financial resources, the dilemma remains. Can central policymakers establish how resources should be used? What is the impact on different client groups? What is the effect on access? In theory, it may well be possible to achieve greater equity in the geographical distribution of resources while inequities among groups or individuals persist or even become worse. But the evidence is strong that there are important differences—linked more to education than to social class—in the ability to make use of health-service facilities.

Therefore a strong case can be made for cross-national studies of the impact of different distributional strategies. The aims of policy seem to be much the same everywhere. But the instruments differ. To what extent does the Finnish PPB system discussed by A. S. Härö help ensure that resources will be devoted to those groups at whom they are aimed? And if they are, can the success of the system be attributed to the sophistication of the financial machinery of control or to the particular kind of relationship that exists between the medical profession and the central government, which is perhaps only possible in a small country? If it is the former, then Finland's innovation should be exportable; if it is the latter, then it may reflect a particular societal situation. Monitoring the effectiveness of various strategies may require information not about the distribution of resources but about the distribution of access. Indeed, one of the main gaps in comparative health service research is our lack of knowledge about the relationship between the distribution of resources and the distribution of access.

The other area in which there appears to be a convergence in innovative experiments is that of health as distinct from medical care. In other words, there is increasing recognition that health services provide social support that may reflect a low or a negligible amount of technical, strictly medical, input. This finding has a number of implications. First, it emphasizes the importance of the organizational relationship between health and other social services. If these services are not only complementary but often interchangeable, what organizational framework can ensure the coordination of policies and day-to-day operations? Second, it stresses the importance of the support provided by the community and raises the question of what factors enhance or diminish the capacity of information networks, such as these discussed by John C. M. Hattinga-Verschure, to provide social support. Finally, it raises the wider issue of the role of national policies—particularly policies concerned with the distribution of incomes and the mobility of labor—in influencing the caring capacity of the community.

In all these fields there is evidence of increasing policy innovation. There is, for example, the Swedish experiment reported in this volume that involves trying to improve coordination between health and other social services. Similar innovations are being tried in Britain and elsewhere. There is the American experiment, described by W. R. Curtis and Duncan Neuhauser, that is concerned with replacing institutional by community-based care in the case of the mentally ill. Similar experiments have taken place in other countries. Finally, many countries have experimented with fiscal measures designed to enhance the ability of families to cope with the disabled, Britain's constant-attendance allowance being only one example among many.

There appears to be great scope for cross-national learning from the success (or failure) of such innovative experiments. But evaluating individual experiments may yield only limited value in the absense of an analytic framework for assessing their applicability or for specifying the precise conditions necessary for their success. If a particular experiment is successful, we need to know the reasons: whether they can be traced to the organizational setting (which may be replicable) or to the social and cultural environment (which cannot be exportable).

Two specific approaches seem to offer a cross-national perspective on innovations. The first relates to whether we can establish, on the basis of examining successful innovations in different countries, the extent to which success depends on scale. Most social innovations designed to enhance cooperation among services or the caring capacity of the community appear to take place in small-scale administrative settings. Do these settings provide a necessary environment for success? If so, there are implications for the organization of health services everywhere. In Britain, for instance, the trend over the past decade has been toward the evolution of large administrative units in the NHS mainly because populations of 200,000 or more appear to offer the most rational way of using expensive *medical* technology. If crossnational studies conclude that large administrative units inhibit the development of a more effective *health*-care support system, then there are strong implications for future policy.

The second issue is the extent to which different systems differ in their capacities to diffuse successful innovations. Although it is interesting to examine and evaluate specific innovative experiments, the crucial question for national policymakers is whether successful experiments can be diffused. The task for crossnational researchers seems to be to ascertain what organizational conditions encourage the diffusion of successful innovations. Health systems may vary in their capacities both to stimulate and to diffuse experimental innovation. One way of analyzing these differences is set forth in Figure 15.1.

Peripheral Incentives and Scope for Innovation		High	Low
	High	Controlled adaptiveness	Pluralistic chaos
	Low	Centralized rigidity	Pluralistic rigidity

Figure 15.1. Central capacity to control the diffusion of innovations.

The United States may be considered an example of pluralistic innovation: extremely successful in stimulating experimental innovation but unsuccessful in controlling its diffusion. Germany may be considered an example of pluralistic rigidity: a variety of administrative levels and a large number of institutions that participate in the implementation of policies discourage local innovation, as suggested by Christa Altenstetter's paper. France may be considered a case of centralized rigidity: The influence of a strong central bureaucracy may discourage peripheral experiment, and the ability to diffuse innovations is circumscribed by a large number of other factors. It is difficult, unfortunately, to find candidates for "Controlled Adaptiveness." Perhaps one of the main challenges in the comparative study of health services may be to ascertain what institutional or organizational factors and patterns of financial incentives conduce to the growth of this category.

REFERENCES

1. OECD Studies in Resource Allocation No. 5. *Public Expenditure Trends.* Paris, June 1978.
2. OECD. *Policies for Innovation in the Service Sector.* Paris, 1977.
3. OECD Studies in Resource Allocation No. 4. *Public Expenditure in Health.* Paris, July 1977.
4. U.S. Congress, Office of Technology Assessment. *Development of Medical Technology.* Washington, August 1976.
5. Glaser, William A. *Paying the Doctor.* Baltimore: Johns Hopkins Press, 1970.
6. Marmor, T. R., and Thomas, D. "Doctors, Politics and Pay Disputes." *British Journal of Political Science,* vol. 2, no. 4, October 1972, 436.
7. Stocking, Barbara, and Morrison, Stuart L. *The Image and the Reality.* London: Oxford University Press, 1978.
8. Office of Health Economics. *Renal Failure,* OHE, April 1978.
9. Buxton, M. J., and Klein, Rudolf. *Allocating Health Resources.* Royal Commission on the National Health Service. Research Paper No. 3. HMSO, 1978.

Bibliography

Abholz, H., et al. "Die Entwicklung der Arbeitermedizin als Beitrag zur Humanisierung der Arbeit." In WSI-Mitteilungen. *IIVG Papers*. 1978/11; RV/78-9.

Alford, Robert R. *Health Care Politics: Ideological and Interest Group Barriers to Reform*. Chicago and London: The University of Chicago Press, 1974.

Alleen samen, *Discussienota over de toekomst van het Kruiswerk*. Utrecht, 1977.

Allgemeine Ortskrankenkasse Amberg. *Geschäftsbericht 1975.*

———. *Geschäftsbericht 1965.*

———. *Geschäfts-und Rechnungsergebnisse 1955.*

———. *Satzung der AOK Amberg.*

Allgemeine Ortskrankenkasse Brilon in Olsberg. *Geschäftsbericht,* für die Jahre 1972–1977.

Allgemeine Ortskrankenkasse Düsseldorf. *Bericht über die Untersuchung der Verwaltungskosten der AOK Düsseldorf,* January 1977.

———. *Bericht über die Untersuchung der Verwaltungskosten des Jahres 1976.*

———. *Satzung der AOK Düsseldorf.*

Allgemeine Ortskrankenkasse Hochsauerlandkreis. *Haushaltsplan für das Haushaltsjahr 1979.*

Allgemeine Ortskrankenkasse Siegerland-Wittgenstein. *Das Geschäftsjahr 1977.*

———. *Das Geschäftsjahr 1976.*

———. *Satzung der AOK Siegerland-Wittgenstein.*

Allgemeine Ortskrankenkasse München. *Statistischer Bericht für das Jahr 1977.*

———. *Geschäftsbericht 1967–1971.*

———. *Geschäftsbericht 1957–1966.*

———. *Organisationsplan.*

———. *Satzung. Stand 1. Januar 1978.*

Allgemeine Ortskrankenkasse Weiden i.d. OPf. *Haushaltsplan mit Erläuterungen für das Geschäftsjahr 1979.*

———. *Geschäftsbericht 1977.*

———. *Satzung.*

Altman, S. H., and Wallack, S. S. "Technology on Trial—Is It the Culprit Behind Rising Health Costs? The Case for and Against." Paper presented at the Sun Valley Forum on National Health, Sun Valley, Idaho, August 1–5, 1977.

American Biology Council. *Contributions of the Biological Sciences to Human Welfare.* Federation Proceedings, vol. 31, 1972.

Arnstein, S. R. "Technology Assessment: Opportunities and Obstacles." In *IEEE Transactions on Systems, Man and Cybernetics* (SMC) 7: 571, 1977.

Ashford, N. *Crisis in the Work Place.* Cambridge, Mass.: MIT Press, 1976.

Banta, H. D., and Bauman, P. "Health Services Research and Health Policy." *Comm. Health* 2: 121, 1976.

Banta, H. D.; Brown, S.; and Behney, D. "Implications of the 1976 Medical Devices Legislation." In *Man and Medicine,* forthcoming.

Banta, H. D., and Sanes, J. R. "Assessing the Social Impacts of Medical Technologies." *J. Comm. Health* 3: 245, 1978.

———. "How the CAT Got out of the Bag." Paper presented at the Conference on Health-Care Technology and the Quality of Care. Boston University Health Policy Center, Boston, Mass., November 19–20, 1976.

Banta, R. F., and Fox, R. C. "Role Strains of a Health Care Team in a Poverty Community." *Soc. Sci. & Med.* 6 (1972): 697–722.

Baram, M. "Medical Device Legislation and the Development and Diffusion of Health Technology." Paper presented at the Conference on Health-Care Technology and the Qualtity of Care, Boston University Health Policy Center, Boston, Mass., November 19–20, 1976.

Bardach, Eugene. *The Implementation Game: What Happens After a Bill Becomes a Law.* Cambridge, Mass.: MIT Press, 1977.

Barnes, S., et al. "Mass Screening for Cancer of the Breast." *Lancet* 1 (1968): 1417.

Battelle Columbus Laboratories. "Analysis of Selected Biomedical Research Programs." In *Report of the President's Biomedical Research Panel.* Washington, D.C.: Department of Health, Education and Welfare, 1976. App. B, p. 35 (DHEW Publications no. OS 75-502).

Becker, Selwyn, and Gordon, Gerald. "An Entrepreneurial Theory of Formal Organizations. Part I: Patterns of Formal Organizations." *Administrative Science Quarterly* 2 (Dec. 1966): 315–334.

Beernink, W. A. M. "Gespreksgroepen met familieleden van verpleeghuisbewoners," no. 8. Netherlands: *Tijdschrift voor Gerontologie,* 1977.

Bennett, I. "Technology as a Shaping Force." *Daedalus* 106 (1977): 125.

Berfenstam, R., and Smedby, B. "Samverkan mellan medicinsk och social vård." *Socialmedicinsk tidskrift* 53 (1976): 365–372.

Berman, D. "Death on the Job." *Monthly Review Press,* 1979.

Bicknell, W., and Walsh, D. "Certificate of Need: The Massachusetts Experience." *N.E.J.M.* 292 (1975).

Biomedical Science and Its Administration. The "Wooldridge Report." Washington, D.C.: The White House, February 1965.

Black, D. "What Should Now Be Done by Government?" *Proc. Roy. Soc. Med.* 67 (1974).

Blanpain, J., and Delesie, L. *Community Health Investment, Health Services Research in Belgium, France, Federal German Republic and the Netherlands.* London: Oxford University Press, 1976.

Blanpain, J., et al. *International Approaches to Health Resources Development for National Health Programs, Executive Summary of the Study.* Hyattsville, Md.: Health Resources Administration, Department of Health, Education and Welfare, 1976.

Blumstein, J. "The Role of PSROs in Hospital Cost Containment." In *Hospital Cost Containment: Selected Notes for Future Policy,* ed. M. Zubkoff, I. Raskin, and R. Hanft. New York: Prodist, 1978.

Boyd, E., et al. "Chromosome Breakage and Ultrasound." *British Medical Journal* 2 (1971): 501.

Breslow, L. *Testimony on Basic Issues in Biomedical Research Before the U.S. Senate Subcommittee on Health, Committee on Labor and Public Welfare.* Washington, D.C., June 17, 1976.

Bronzino, J. D. *Technology for Patient Care.* St. Louis: C. V. Mosby Co., 1977.

Brotherston, J. "Inequality: Is It Inevitable?" In *Equalities and Inequalities in Health,* ed. C. Carter and J. Peel. London: Academic Press, 1977.

Brown, S. S. *Policy Issues in the Health Sciences.* Washington, D.C.: Institute of Medicine, National Academy of Sciences, 1977.

Bundesverband der Ortskrankenkassen. *Die Ortskrankenkassen, 1975.*

Bunker, J. P.; Barnes, B. A.; and Mosteller, F., eds. *Costs, Risks, and Benefits of Surgery.* New York: Oxford University Press, 1977.

Buxton, M. J., and Klein, Rudolf. *Allocating Health Resources.* Research Paper no. 3, Royal Commission on the National Health Service. London: HMSO, 1978.

Carlson, Rick. *The End of Medicine.* New York: John Wiley and Sons, 1975.

Carmichael, J. H. E., and Berry, R. J. "Diagnostic X-rays in Late Pregnancy and in the Reonate." *Lancet* 1 (1976).

Carter, C., and Peel, J., eds. *Equalities and Inequalities in Health.* London: Academic Press, 1977.

Chamberlain, J., et al. "Validity of Clinical Examination and Mammography as Screening Tests for Breast Cancer." *Lancet* 2 (1975).

Cochrane, A. L. *Effectiveness and Efficiency: Random Reflections on Health Services.* London: Burgess & Son Ltd (Nuffield Provincial Hospitals Trust), 1972.

———. "Some Reflections." In *A Question of Quality? Roads to Assurance in Medical Care,* ed. G. McLachlan. London: Oxford University Press, 1976.

Comroe, J. H. "Lags Between Initial Discovery and Clinical Application to Cardiovascular Pulmonary Medicine and Surgery." In *Report of the President's Biomedical Research Panel.* Washington, D.C.: Department of Health, Education and Welfare, 1976.

Council on Wage and Price Stability. *The Complex Puzzle of Rising Health Care Costs: Can the Private Sector Fit It Together?* Washington, D.C.: Executive Office of the President, 1976.

Cour des Comptes. "Rapport au Président de la République." *Journal Officiel,* 2 July 1977.

Cromwell, J. *Evaluation of Effects of Certificate of Need Programs.* Contract no. HRA 231-77-0114, National Center for Health Services Research. Rockville, Md.: Department of Health, Education and Welfare, 1977.

Cromwell, J., et al. *Incentives and Decisions Underlying Hospitals' Adoption and Utilization of Major Capital Equipment.* Boston, Mass.: Abt Associates, Inc., 1975.

Crossman, Richard. *Diaries of a Cabinet Minister,* vol. 3, 1968–1977. London: Hamish Hamilton and Jonathan Cape, 1977.

Curtis, W. Robert. "Area Strategy." *Social Matrix Research Publications Series.* Boston, Mass., 1978.

———. "Community Human Service Networks: New Roles for Mental Health Workers." *Psychiatric Annals,* vol. 3, no. 7 (July 1973).

———. "From State Hospital to Integrated Human Service System." *Health Care Management Review,* vol. 1, no. 2 (Spring 1976).

———. "Team Problem Solving in a Social Network." *Psychiatric Annals,* vol. 4, no. 12 (December 1974).

———. "The Clinical Trial: A Study of Social Network and Clinical Intervention." Ph.D. dissertation, Harvard School of Public Health, 1978.

———. "What Follows Services Integration? Simulated Decentralized State Organizations Delivering Comprehensive Human Services." Boston, Mass.: Social Matrix Research, Inc., 1977.

Curtis, W. Robert, and Neuhauser, Duncan. "Providing Specialized Coordinated Human

Services to Communities: The Organizational Problem and a Potential Solution." Position Paper no. 4, *Ford Foundation Seminar on the Delivery of Urban Health Services.* Boston, Mass.: Harvard School of Public Health.

Davis, Stanley, and Lawrence, Paul. *Matrix.* Reading, Mass.: Addison-Wesley Publishing Co., 1977.

De Haen, P. "The Drug Lag—Does It Exist in Europe?" *Drug Intelligence and Clinical Pharmacy* 9 (1975).

De Haes, W. F. M.; Schuurman, J. H.; and Sturmans, F. "Gezondheidsvoorlichting-en opvoeding. Gedragsdeterminaten." *Medisch Contact* 31 (1976).

Department of Health, Education and Welfare. *Forward Plan for Health, FY 1978–1982.* Washington, D.C.: U.S. Government Printing Office, 1976.

———. *Health, United States, 1976–1977.* Washington, D.C.: U.S. Government Printing Office, 1977.

———. "National Guidelines for Health Planning." *Federal Register* 43 (March 28, 1978).

———. *Papers on the National Health Guidelines: Baselines for Setting Health Goals and Standards.* DHEW Publication no. HRA 76-640. Washington, D.C.: U.S. Government Printing Office, 1976.

Department of Health and Social Service. *DHSS Planning Guidelines for 1978–1979.* Circular HC(78)12, March 1978.

———. *Priorities for Health and Personal Social Services in England.* London: HMSO, 1976.

———. *Report of the Supply Board Working Group.* London: HMSO, May 1978.

———. *The Way Forward.* London: HMSO, 1977.

Dunham, Andrew B., and Marmor, Theodore R. "Federal Policy and Health: Recent Trends and Different Perspectives," pp. 263–298. In *Nationalizing Government: Public Policies in America,* ed. Theodore J. Lowi and Alan Stone. Beverly Hills and London: Sage Publications, 1978.

Ellwood, Paul. "Restructuring the Health Delivery System." In *Health Maintenance Organizations: A Reconfiguration of the Health Services System.* Proceedings of the Thirteenth Annual Symposium on Hospital Affairs, University of Chicago, Chicago, Ill., May 1971.

Enthoven, Alain. "Consumer Choice Health Plan: An Approach to National Health Insurance Based on Regulated Competition in the Private Sector." Proposed NHI Plan and Its Central Role for HMOs. Paper presented to HEW Secretary Joseph Califano, September 1977.

Faure, H.; Sandier, S.; and Tonnelier, F. "Analyse régionale des relations entre l'offre et la consommation de soins médicaux (secteur privé). *CREDOC.*

Fineberg, H. N. "Gastric Freezing, A Study of Diffusion of a Medical Innovation." Paper prepared for the Committee on Technology and Health Care, National Academy of Sciences, Washington, D.C., August 1977.

Finkel, M. "FDA Implementing Plans To Cut by One or Two Years New-Drug Approval Lag." *Medical Tribune* 14 (1973).

Fisher, B. "Primary Therapy of Breast Cancer: A Report," pp. 157–170. In *Report to the Profession—Breast Cancer.* Washington, D.C.: National Cancer Institute, National Institutes of Health, 1974.

Fletcher, E. W. L. "Is Foetal Radiography Really Necessary?" *Lancet* 1 (1978).

Freeman, C. "Economics of Research and Development." In *Science Technology and Society,* ed. I. Spiegel-Rösing and D. Price. London: Sage Publications, 1977.

Fuchs, V. "The Growing Demand for Medical Care." *N.E.J.M.* 279 (1968).

———. "Health Care and the U.S. Economic System, An Essay in Abnormal Physiology." *Milbank Mem. Fund Quart. L.* 211 (1972).

Gardner, A., and Riessman, F. *Self-help in the Human Services.* Jossey-Bass, 1977.

Gaus, C. R., and Cooper, B. S. "Controlling Health Technology." Paper presented at the Sun Valley Forum on National Health, Sun Valley, Idaho, August 1–5, 1977.

———. "Technology and Medicare: Alternatives for Change." Paper presented at the Conference on Health-Care Technology and the Quality of Care, Boston University Health Policy Center, Boston, Mass., November 19–20, 1976.

Gaus, G. "Biomedical Research and Health Care Costs." Testimony Before the President's Biomedical Research Panel. Washington, D.C., September 29, 1975.

Gehan, E., and Freireich, E. "Nonrandomized Control in Cancer Clinical Trials." *N.E.J.M.* 290 (1974).

Gibson, R. M., and Mueller, M. S. "National Health Expenditures, Fiscal Year 1976." *Social Security Bulletin* 40 (1977): 3–22.

Gillick, Muriel. "The Criteria of Choice in Medical Policy: Radiotherapy." *Massachusetts Minerva* 15 (Spring 1977): 15–31.

Gilmore, M.; Bruce, N.; and Hunt, M. *The Work of the Nursing Team in General Practice.* London: Council for the Education and Training of Health Visitors, 1974.

Glaser, William A. *Paying the Doctor.* Baltimore: Johns Hopkins Press, 1970.

Gordon, G., and Fisher, G. L., eds. *The Diffusion of Medical Technology.* Cambridge, Mass.: Ballinger Publishing Co., 1975.

The Government's Expenditure Plans, 1978–1979 to 1981–1982. London: HMSO, 1976.

Grabowski, H., and Vernon, J. M. "Innovation and Invention, Consumer Protection Regulations in Ethical Drugs." *American Economic Association. Proceedings of Annual Meeting* 67 (1976).

Grabowski, H.; Vernon, J. M.; and Thomas, L. G. "The Effects of Regulatory Policy on the Incentives to Innovate: International Comparative Analysis." Paper presented before the Third Seminar on Pharmaceutical Public Policy Issues, College of Public Affairs, American University, Washington, D.C., December 15, 1975.

Greer, A. L. *Hospital Adoption of Medical Technology: A Preliminary Investigation into Hospital Decision Making.* Milwaukee, Wis.: The University of Wisconsin–Milwaukee, Urban Research Center, 1977.

Grelot, Jean-Philippe, and Soufflet, Hervé. "L'insuffisance rénale chronique: analyse comparée de la dialyse et la transplantation." Assistance Publique de Paris: Centre de Recherche en Gestion, Ecole Polytechnique, January 1977.

Griliches, Z. "Research Costs and Social Returns: Hybrid Corn and Related Innovations." *Journal of Political Economy* (October 1958).

Hakkarainen, A. *Introducing Primary Health Services on a Nationwide Scale* (DSTI/SPR/75.60/22B). Paris: Organization for Economic Cooperation and Development, 1977.

Hattinga-Verschure, J. C. M. "Ontwikkeling van zorgcriteria voor herstructurering van de gezondheidszorg." *Het ziekenhuis* 2 (1972).

———. *Het verschijnsel zorg.* Lochem, Neth.: De Tijdstroom, 1977.

Hauss, F., and Naschold, F. "Arbeitsschutz und Sozialpartnerschaft in Schweden: Informationen und Thesen." *IIVG Papers.* Berlin: WZB; October 1978.

Haverkamp, A. D., et al. "The Evaluation of Continuous Fetal Heart Rate Monitoring in High-Risk Pregnancy." *Am. J. Obstet. Gynecol.* 125 (1976).

Havighurst, C. "Controlling Health Care Costs: Strengthening the Private Sector's Hand." *Health Politics, Policy, and Law* 1 (Winter 1977): 471–498.

———. "Federal Regulation of the Health Care Delivery System: A Foreword in the Nature of a 'Package Insert.' " *University of Toledo Law Review* 6 (1975).

Health Services Administration. *Professional Standards Review Organizations: Program Evaluation, Executive Summary.* Washington, D.C.: Department of Health, Education and Welfare, October 1977.

Hellinger, F. J. "The Effect of Certificate-of-Need Legislation on Hospital Investment." *Inquiry* 13 (1976).

Herskowitz, Julia, and Curtis, W. Robert. "Deinstitutionalization and Its Effects on Employees." *Social Matrix Research Monograph Publication Series*. Boston, Mass., 1977.

———. "The Psychiatric Hospital Employee: A Resource for Social Change." *Health Care Management Review,* 2 (Winter 1977).

Hiatt, H. H. "Protecting the Medical Commons: Who Is Responsible?" *N.E.J.M.* 293 (1975).

Hilton, G. "The Basic Behavior of Regulatory Commissions." *American Economic Review* (May 1972): 47–54.

Hunt, Audrey. *The Elderly at Home*. London: HMSO, 1978.

Huygen, F. J. A. *Waar gaat onze gezondheidszorg naar toe*. Bilthoven: Ambo, 1977.

Iglehart, J. K. "The Cost and Regulation of Medical Technology: Future Policy Directions." *Milbank Mem. Fund Q.* 55 (1977).

Improving Health Care Through Research and Development, Report of the Panel on Health Services Research and Development of the President's Science Advisory Committee. Washington, D.C.: U.S. Government Printing Office, 1972.

Institute of Medicine. *A Policy Statement: Computer Tomographic Scanning*. Washington, D.C.: National Academy of Sciences, April 1977.

Investigation of the National Institutes of Health, Prepared by the Staff for the Use of the Committee on Interstate and Foreign Commerce, U.S. House of Representatives. Washington, D.C.: U.S. Government Printing Office, 1976.

Johnson, Lyndon B. *The Vantage Point: Perspectives on the Presidency, 1963–1969*. New York: Holt, Rinehart and Winston, 1971.

Jonsson, E., and Marke, L. A. "Computer Assisted Tomography of the Head." Economic Analysis for Sweden, Stockholm, Sweden. *SPRI*. July 1976.

Kaluzny, A. D. "Innovation in Health Services, Theoretical Framework and Review of Research." *Health Serv. Res.* 9 (1974).

Kaluzny, A. D.; Veney, J. E.; and Gentry, J. T. "Innovation of Health Services: A Comparative Study of Hospitals and Health Departments." *MMFQ/Health and Society* 52 (1974).

Kaprio, L. "The Health Care Picture of Europe." DHEW Publication no. HRA 76-638. In *Health Services Systems in the European Economic Community*. Hyattsville, Md.: Health Resources Administration, Department of Health, Education and Welfare, 1975.

Kervasdoué, Jean de. "Power, Efficiency and Adoption of Innovations in Formal Organizations." Ph.D. dissertation, Cornell University, 1973.

Kervasdoué, Jean de, and Billow, François. "Developpement de la recherche et influences externes: Le cas du cancer et des affections respiratoires." Paris: Centre de Recherche en Gestion, Ecole Polytechnique, Janvier 1978.

Kervasdoué, Jean de, and Kimberly, John. "Are Organizational Structures Culture Free: The Case of Hospital Innovations in the U.S. and France." Paper presented at the Conference on Crosscultural Studies on Organizational Functioning, Honolulu, Hawaii, September, 1977.

Klein, Rudolf. "The Corporate State, the Health Service and the Professions." *New University Quarterly* 31 (Spring 1972).

———. "The Rise and Decline of Policy Analysis: The Strange Case of Health Policymaking in Britain." *Policy Analysis* 2 (1976).

Kohn, R. "Coordination of Health and Welfare Services in Four Countries: Austria, Italy, Poland, and Sweden." *Public Health in Europe*. 6. Copenhagen: Regional Office for Europe, World Health Organization, 1977.

Kühn, H., and Hauss, F. "Entwicklungstendenzen im medizinischen Arbeitsschutz: Thesen," PV/78-5. *IIVG Papers*. West Berlin: WZB, May 1978. Reprinted in Jahrbuch für Kritische Medizin, Argument. West Berlin: Sonderband, 1978.

Kuiper, J. P. *Het zal onze zorg zijn*. Assen/Amsterdam: Van Gorcum, 1978.

Lacronique, Jean-François. "Cross-sectional International Analysis of the Consumption of

Short-term Medical Care." Master's thesis, Massachusetts Institute of Technology, June 1977.

Lalonde, M. "A New Perspective on the Health of Canadians." Ottawa: Government of Canada, 1974.

Landstingsforbundet, Svenska Kommunförbundet, Socialstyrelsen och SPRI. *Primärvård Aldreomsorger Samverkan.* Stockholm, 1977.

Lasagna, L. "Research, Regulation, and Development of New Pharmaceuticals: Past, Present, and Future." *Am. J. Med. Sci.* 263 (1972).

Laurence, K. M. "Screening for Disease: Foetal Malformations and Abnormalities." *Lancet* 2 (1974).

De leefsituatie van de Nederlandse bevolking 1974. *Deel 1: kerncijfers.* 's-Gravenhage: Staatsuitgeverij, 1975.

Le Gall, Jean-René. "Le profil du coût des santés." Mimeographed, Paris, 1977.

Leighton, P. C., et al. "Levels of Alpha-fetoprotein in Maternal Blood as a Screening Test for Fetal Neural Tube Defects." *Lancet* 2 (1975).

Lewin & Associates. *Government Controls on the Health Care System: The Canadian Experience.* Washington, D.C.: Lewin & Associates, 1976.

Lindblom, C. E. "The Science of 'Muddling Through.' " *Publ. Adm. Rev.* 19 (1959): 79–99.

Arthur D. Little and Industrial Research Institute. *Barriers to Innovation in Industry: Opportunities for Public Policy Changes.* National Science Foundation Contracts no. NSF-C748 and C725. Washington, D.C.: Arthur D. Little, 1973.

Lowi, Theodore J., and Stone, Alan, eds. *Nationalizing Government: Public Policies in America.* Beverly Hills and London: Sage Publications, 1978.

McKeown, T. "A Historical Appraisal of the Medical Task." In *Medical History and Medical Care,* ed. G. McLachlan and T. McKeown. New York: Oxford University Press, 1971.

———. *The Role of Medicine: Dream, Mirage, or Nemesis.* London: Nuffield Prov. Hospitals Trust, 1976.

McLachlan, G. *Challenges for Change, Essays on the Next Decade in the National Health Services.* London: Oxford University Press, 1971.

———. *Measuring for Management: Quantitative Methods in Health Service Management.* London: Oxford University Press, 1975.

———. *Positions, Movements and Directions in Health Services Research.* London: Oxford University Press, 1974.

———. *A Question of Quality: Roads to Assurance in Medical Care.* London: Oxford University Press, 1976.

Mahler, H. "Blueprint for Health for All." *WHO Chronicle* 31 (1977): 491–498.

———. "Health–A Demystification of Medical Technology." *Lancet* 2 (1975).

Mansfield, E. *Economics of Technological Change.* New York, 1968.

Mansfield, E., et al. *Research and Innovation in the Modern Corporation.* New York: W. W. Norton & Co., 1971.

March, James, and Simon, Herbert. *Organizations.* New York: John Wiley and Sons, 1958.

Marmor, T. R., and Thomas, D. "Doctors, Politics and Pay Disputes." *British Journal of Political Science,* vol. 2, no. 1 (October 1972).

Maxwell, R. *Health Care, the Growing Dilemma, Needs Versus Resources in Western Europe, the US and the USSR.* A McKinsey Survey Report. London: McKinsey & Co., Inc., 1975.

Mechanic, D. "The Growth of Medical Technology and Bureaucracy: Implications for Medical Care." *MMFO/Health and Society* 55 (1977).

———. *Public Expectations and Health Care.* New York: John Wiley–Interscience (John Wiley and Sons), 1972.

Meire, H. B. "Radiology Now: Ultrasound–Current Status and Prospects." *British Journal of Radiology* 50 (1977).

Naschold, F. "Arbeitsschutz in den USA und präventive Sozialpolitik," dp-78/17. Internationales Institut für Vergleichende Gesellschaftsforschung. West Berlin: Wissenschaftszentrum Berlin, October 1978. Reprinted in *WSI-Mitteilungen,* 1978/10.

National Academy of Sciences. *Medical Technology and the Health Care System: A Study of Equipment-Embodied Technology.* Washington, D.C.: The National Research Council and the Institute of Medicine, 1978.

The National Board of Health and Welfare. *The Tierp Project—Its Objectives, Organization, and Fields of Activity.* Stockholm, 1977.

National Health Service Act, 1977. London: HMSO, 1977.

National Health Service Reorganisation: England. Cmnd. 5055. London: HMSO, 1972.

National Institutes of Health. *Inventory of Clinical Trials, Fiscal Year 1975.* Bethesda, Md.: Division of Research Grants, National Institutes of Health, 1977.

———. *The Responsibilities of NIH at the Health Research/Health Care Interface.* Report of the Office of the Director. Bethesda, Md.: National Institutes of Health, February 14, 1977.

The National Swedish Board of Health and Welfare. *The Swedish Health Services in the 1980s.* Stockholm, 1976.

Neuhauser, D., and Jonsson, E. "Managerial Response to New Health Care Technology: Coronary Artery Bypass Surgery." In *The Management of Health Care,* ed. W. J. Abernathy, A. Sheldon, and C. K. Prahalad. Cambridge, Mass.: Ballinger Publishing Co., 1974.

Noll, R. G. "The Consequences of Public Utility Regulation of Hospitals." In Institute of Medicine, *Control of Health Care.* Washington, D.C.: National Academy of Sciences, 1975.

Novick, D., and Euthoven, A. "Long-Range Planning Through Program Budgeting." In *Perspectives of Planning,* ed. E. Jantsch. Paris: Organization for Economic Cooperation and Development, 1969.

Office of Health Economics. *Renal Failure.* OHE, April 1978.

Office of Population Censuses and Survey. *The General Household Survey: Introductory Report.* London: HMSO, 1973 and subsequent.

Office of Technology Assessment. *Assessing the Efficacy and Safety of Medical Technologies.* Washington, D.C.: U.S. Government Printing Office, September 1978.

———. *Development of Medical Technology: Opportunities for Assessment.* Washington, D.C.: U.S. Government Printing Office, 1976.

Organization for Economic Cooperation and Development. *Changing Priorities for Government R&D.* Paris: Organization for Economic Cooperation and Development, 1975.

———. *Dépensées publiques de Santé.* Paris: OECD, February 1977.

———. *Policies for Innovation in the Service Sector.* Paris: OECD, 1977.

———. *Studies in Resource Allocation, no. 4. Public Expenditure in Health.* Paris: OECD, July 1977.

———. *Studies in Resource Allocation, no. 5. Public Expenditure Trends.* Paris: OECD, June 1978.

Paradise, J. L. "Pittsburgh Tonsillectomy and Adenoidectomy Study: Differences from Earlier Studies and Problems of Execution." *Ann. Otol. Rhinol. Laryngol.* 84 (1975).

Peltzman, S. *Regulation of Pharmaceutical Innovation, the 1962 Amendments.* Washington, D.C.: American Enterprise Institute for Public Policy Research, 1974.

Perrow, Charles. "Hospitals: Technology, Structure, and Goals." In *Handbook of Organizations,* ed. James G. March. Chicago: Rand McNally, 1965.

Policy Implications of the Computed Tomography (CT) Scanner. Washington, D.C.: U.S. Government Printing Office, August 1978.

President's Biomedical Research Panel. *Report of the President's Biomedical Research Panel.* DHEW no. OS 76-500. Washington, D.C.: U.S. Department of Health, Education and Welfare, April 30, 1976.

Preston, T. A. *Coronary Artery Surgery: A Critical Review.* New York: Raven Press, 1977.

Puro, Karl. "Our Health" (Kansanterveytemme). H. S., 20, 22, and 25 October 1971.

Rapoport, J. *Diffusion of Technological Innovation in Hospitals: A Case Study of Nuclear Medicine.* Photocopy. South Hadley, Mass., 1976.

Reed, M. F. "Ultrasonic Placentography." *British Journal of Radiology* 46 (1973).

Registrar General. *Occupational Mortality, 1970–1972.* London: OPCS, HMSO, 1978.

Reijners, B., et al. "Wie zorgt daarvoor? Een oriënterend onderzoek naar aanknopingspunten voor weizijnsverbetering." In *Verpleeghuis Vreugdehof Amsterdam. Report.* Utrecht: Institute of Hospital Sciences, 1978.

Reinhardt, U. E. *National Health Insurance in Australia, Canada, France, West Germany, and the Netherlands: A Synopsis.* Prepared for the National Center for Health Services Research. International Workshop on Health Insurance, September 25–27, 1977.

The Relationship of Expenditure to Needs. Eighth Report of the Expenditure Committee for 1971–1972, HC 575. London: HMSO, 1972.

Renaud, Marc. "Reforme ou illusion? Une analyse des interventions de l'Etat quebecois dans le domaine de la santé." *Sociologie et Sociétés* 9 (Avril 1977).

Report of the Committee on the Economic and Financial Problems of the Provision for Old Age, Cmd. 9333. London: HMSO, 1954.

Rettig, R. A. *Cancer Crusade: The Story of the National Cancer Act of 1971.* Princeton, N.J.: Princeton University Press, 1977.

Rettig, R. A.; Sorg, J. D.; and Milward, H. B. *Criteria for the Allocation of Resources to Research and Development: A Review of the Literature.* Washington, D.C.: National Science Foundation, 1974.

Riveline, C. "Esquisse d'une nouvelle économie d'entreprise." *Annales des Mines,* Avril 1977.

Robb, Barbara, ed. *Sans Everything: A Case to Answer.* London: Nelson, 1967.

Roemer, M. I. "Regulation in Different Types of Health Care Systems." In *Health Care Systems in World Perspective,* ed. M. I. Roemer. Ann Arbor, Mich.: Health Administrative Press, 1976.

Rogers, David E. "The Challenge of Primary Care." *Daedalus* (Winter 1977).

Rogers, E. M., and Shoemaker, F. F. *Communication of Innovations, A Crosscultural Approach.* New York: The Free Press, 1971.

Rothenberg, E. *Regulation and Expansion of Health Facilities: The Certificate of Need Experience in New York State.* New York: Praeger, 1978.

Rothschild (Lord). *A Framework for Government Research and Development.* London: HMSO, 1971.

Rouwenhorst. W. *Leren gezond te zijn?* Alphen a/d Rijn: Samson, 1977.

Rubin, I. M., and Beckhard, R. "Factors Influencing the Effectiveness of Health Teams." *Milbank Mem. Fund Q.* 50 (1972): 317–335, Part 1.

Russell, L. B. "The Diffusion of New Hospital Technologies in the United States." *International Journal of Health Services* 6 (1976).

———. "Making Rational Decisions About Medical Technology." Paper presented before the American Medical Association's National Commission on the Cost of Medical Care. Chicago, Ill., November 23, 1976.

Sadler, Judith. "Ideologies of 'Art' and 'Science' in Medicine: The Transition from Medical Care to the Application of Technique in the British Medical Profession." Memorandum, University of Manchester, 1977.

Salkever, D. S. "Will Regulation Control Health Care Costs?" *Bulletin of the New York Academy of Medicine* 54 (January 1978): 73–83.

Salkever, D. S., and Bice, T. W. "The Impact of Certificate-of-Need Controls on Hospital Investment." *Milbank Memorial Fund Quarterly/Health and Society* (Spring 1976): 185–214.

———. "Certificate-of-Need Legislation and Hospital Costs." In *Hospital Cost Contain-*

ment: Selected Notes for Future Policy, ed. M. Zubkoff; I. E. Raskin; and R. S. Hanft. New York: Prodist, 1978.

Schifrin, L. G., and Tayan, J. R. "The Drug Lag: An Interpretive Review of the Literature." *Int. J. Health Serv.* 7 (1977).

Schmookler, J. *Invention and Economic Growth.* Cambridge, Mass.: Harvard University Press, 1966.

Schroeder, S. A., and Showstack, J. A. "The Dynamics of Medical Technology Use: Analysis and Policy Options." Paper presented at the Sun Valley Forum on National Health, Sun Valley, Idaho, August 1–5, 1977.

Schuurman, J. H.; de Haes, W. F. M.; and Sturmans, F. "Verandering van gedrag." *Medisch Contact* 31 (1976).

———. "Opvoeding tot gezond gedrag." *Medisch Contact* 31 (1976).

Scitovsky, A. A. "Changes in Treatment and the Costs of 'Common' Illness." Paper presented at the Sun Valley Forum on National Health, Sun Valley, Idaho, August 1–5, 1977.

Sedeuilh, M. "Requirements and Data Availability for Health Care Systems in Europe." In *Proceedings of an International Conference on Health Technology Systems, San Francisco.* Potomac, Md.: Health Applications Section, Operations Research Society of America, 1974.

Shepard, D. *Analysis of Biomedical Research, Fourth Aspect of Task, An Analysis of How New Technology Is Diffused Throughout the Health Care System.* Report prepared for the Office of Health Policy Analysis and Research, Department of Health, Education and Welfare, August 29, 1973.

Sherman, H. "Research, Development and Innovation in Health Care Organizations." In *The Management of Health Care,* ed. W. J. Abernathy, A. Sheldon, and C. K. Prahalad. Cambridge, Mass.: Ballinger Publishing Co., 1974.

Simmons, H. E. "The Drug Regulatory System of the United States Food and Drug Administration: A Defense of Current Requirements for Safety and Efficacy." *Int. J. Health Serv.* 4 (1974).

Socialstyrelsen. *Samarbete mellan socialvård samt hälsooch sjukvård.* Stockholm, 1977.

Spending on the Health and Personal Social Services. Ninth Report of the Expenditure Committee for 1976–1977, HC 466. London: HMSO, 1977.

Spingarn, N. D. *Heartbeat: The Politics of Health Research.* Washington, D.C.: Robert B. Luce, 1976.

Spitz, Bruce. "Medicaid Cost Containment Policy: HMO Regulation and Reimbursement," Working paper. Washington, D.C.: The Urban Institute, April 1977.

———. *Paper Submitted to HEW Secretary Joseph Califano.* September 1977.

Starr, Paul. "Medicine and the Waning of Professional Sovereignty." Paper prepared for the Daedalus Conference, January 28–29, 1977.

Stephan, Jean-Claude. *Economie et Pouvoir Médical.* Paris: Economica édit., 1978.

Stewart, A., and Kneale, G. W. "Changes in the Cancer Risk Associated with Radiology." *Lancet* 1 (1968).

Stigler, G. J. "The Theory of Economic Regulation." *Bell Journal of Economics and Management Science* 2 (Spring 1971).

Strickland, S. P. *Politics, Science, and Dread Disease.* Cambridge, Mass.: Harvard University Press, 1972.

Stocking, Barbara, and Morrison, Stuart L. *The Image and the Reality.* London: Oxford University Press, 1978.

Tennstedt, Florian. *Soziale Selbstverwaltung.* Band 2, Bonn: Verlag der Ortskrankenkassen, 1977.

Thomas, L. "Aspects of Biomedical Science Policy." Address to the Institute of Medicine, Fall Meeting. Occasional Papers of the Institute of Medicine. Washington, D.C.: National Academy of Sciences, 1972.

———. *The Lives of a Cell.* New York: The Viking Press, 1974.

———. "On the Science and Technology of Medicine." *Daedalus* (Winter 1977).

Töns, Hans. *Grundausbildung für den Krankenkassendienst.* Sankt Augustin: Asgard Verlag, 12. überarbeitete Auflage, Juli 1980.

Van Langendonck, J. "Social Health Insurance in the E. E. C." In *Health Services Systems in the European Community.* DHEW Publication no. HRA 76-638. Hyattsville, Md.: Health Resources Administration, Department of Health, Education and Welfare, 1975.

"The Veterans Administration Cooperative Randomized Study of Surgery for Coronary Arterial Occlusive Disease." *Circulation* 54 (December 1976, Supp. 3).

"The Veterans Administration Cooperative Study Group on Antihypertensive Agents." *J.A.M.A.* 202 (1967) and *J.A.M.A.* 213 (1970).

von Ferber, Christian and Bogs, H. *Soziale Selbstverwaltung.* Band 1, Bonn: Verlag der Ortskrankenkassen, 1977.

Wagner, J. L., and Zubkoff, M. "Medical Technology and Hospital Costs." In *Hospital Cost Containment: Selected Notes for Future* Policy, ed. M. Zubkoff; I. E. Raskin; and R. S. Hanft. New York: Prodist, 1978.

Waldman, S. *The Effect of Changing Technology on Hospital Costs.* Research and Statistics Note no. 4–1972. Washington, D.C.: Office of Research and Statistics, Social Security Administration, February 28, 1972.

Ward, G. M. *Memorandum from the National High Blood Pressure Education Program, National Institutes of Health, to the Office of Technology Assessment.* Washington, D.C., January 18, 1977.

Wardell, W. M. "British Usage and American Awareness of Some New Therapeutic Drugs." *Clin. Pharmacol. Ther.* 14 (1973).

———. "Introduction of New Therapeutic Drugs in the United States and Great Britain: An International Comparison." *Clin. Pharmacol. Ther.* 14 (1973).

———. "Therapeutic Implications of the Drug Lag." *Clin. Pharmacol. Ther.* 15 (1974).

Wardell, W. M., and Lasagna, L. *Regulation and Drug Development.* Washington, D.C.: American Enterprise Institute for Public Policy Research, 1975.

Warner, K. E. "The Cost of Capital-Embodied Medical Technology." Paper prepared for the Committee on Technology and Health Care, National Academy of Sciences, July 1977.

———. "A 'Desperation Reaction' Model of Medical Diffusion." *Health Serv. Res.* 10 (1975).

———. "Treatment Decision Making in Catastrophic Illness." *Med. Care* 15 (1977).

Weinberg, A. M. "Criteria for Scientific Choice." *Minerva* 1 (1963).

Weinstein, M. "Allocation of Subjects in Medical Experiments." *N.E.J.M.* 291 (1974).

Wennberg, J. E., and Gittelsohn, A. "Health Care Delivery in Maine: Patterns of Use of Common Surgical Procedures." *J. Maine Med. Assoc.* 66 (1975).

———. "Small Area Variations in Health Care Delivery." *Science* 182 (1973).

White, K. L., and Murnaghan, J. H. "Health Care Policy Formation: Analysis, Information, and Research." *Int. J. Health Serv.* 3 (1973).

Wildavsky, Aaron. "Doing Better and Feeling Worse." *Daedalus* (Winter 1977).

Wiley, J. P. "What's Holding Up New Drug Development?" *FDA Consumer* 7 (1973).

Willems, J., et al. "The Computed Tomography Scanner." Paper presented at the Sun Valley Forum on National Health, Sun Valley, Idaho, August 1–5, 1977.

Willocks, Donald, et. al. "Intrauterine Growth Assessed by Ultrasonic Foetal Cephalometry." *J. Obs. Gyn. Brit. Comm.* 74 (1967).

Wirtschafts- und Sozialwissenschaftliches Institut des Deutschen Gewerkschaftsbundes. *Sozialpolitik und Selbstverwaltung.* Köln: Bund-Verlag, 1977.

World Health Organization. *Development of Health Programme Evaluation.* Thirty-first World Health Assembly, A 31/10. Geneva, WHO, 1978.

———. *Organizational Study on Methods of Promoting the Development of Basic Health Services,* Official Records no. 206. Geneva: WHO, 1973.
———. *World Health Statistics Annual,* vol. 3, *Health Personnel and Hospital Establishments.* Geneva: WHO, 1977.
Young, C. B. "Mammography and Paraclinical Examination of the Breast." In *Recent Advances in Radiology,* ed. T. Lodge and B. E. Steiner. Edinburgh: Churchill, 1975.
Zubkoff, M.; Raskin, I. E.; and Hanft, R. S., eds. *Hospital Cost Containment: Selected Notes for Future Policy.* New York: Prodist, 1978.

Index

A

B

N

O

P

Q

R

S

T

U

About the Science Center Berlin

The Science Center Berlin (Wissenschaftszentrum Berlin), a nonprofit corporation, serves as a parent institution for institutes conducting social science research in areas of significant social concern.

The following institutes are currently operating within the Science Center Berlin:

1. The International Institute of Management,
2. The International Institute for Environment and Society,
3. The International Institute for Comparative Social Research.

They share the following structural elements: a multinational professional and supporting staff, multidisciplinary project teams, a focus on international comparative studies, a policy orientation in the selection of research topics and the diffusion of results.

About the Editor and Contributors

Christa Altenstetter, visiting research fellow at the International Institute of Management in Berlin and associate professor of political science at the City University of New York, received the Ph.D. in political science in 1967 from Heidelberg University. She has taught and/or researched at a number of universities and institutions, including Heidelberg, Harvard, Kiel, Syracuse, Yale, the Urban Institute, and the National Institutes of Health (Fogarty International Center). Dr. Altenstetter has served as a consultant to the U.S. Department of Health, Education and Welfare, the World Health Organization, the National Academy of Sciences, and the Fulbright Hays Commission. Her most recent publications—"Hospital Planning in France and the Federal Republic of Germany," "Health Policy Implementation and Corporate Participation in the Federal Republic of Germany," "Health Planning Methods for Ambulatory Care . . . ," "Hospital Planning in North-Rhine Westfalia . . . ," and *Organizations for Managing Hospital Planning Programs in France and the Federal Republic of Germany*—reflect her research interests in the politics and organization of health planning and implementation processes in comparative perspective. She is editor of a cross-national volume on *Changing National-Subnational Relations in Health: Opportunities and Constraints* and is writing a book on *Health Program Implementation in the Federal Republic of Germany, 1955–1975.*

David Banta, health program manager of the Office of Technology Assessment, Congress of the United States, earned an M.D. degree at Duke University and was trained in public health, preventive medicine, and health-services administration at Harvard University. He was on the community-medicine faculty at Mount Sinai School of Medicine from 1969 to 1974. From 1974 to 1975, Dr. Banta was a Robert Wood Johnson health policy fellow with the Institute of Medicine, National Academy of Sciences, and also worked on the staffs of Senator Jacob Javits and Congressman Paul Rogers. In 1975 he joined the Health Program staff of the Office of Technology Assessment, and in 1978 he became the head of the program. In recent years Dr. Banta has focused on the benefits, risks, and costs of medical technology from a policy perspective, helping develop programs to ensure the adequate assessment of medical technologies. He has also worked on specific technologies, particularly computed tomography (CT) scanning and electronic fetal monitoring.

Ragnar Berfenstam received his medical education at the University of Uppsala, Sweden, graduating in 1943. Thereafter he specialized in pediatrics at Uppsala, where he was appointed assistant professor in pediatrics in 1952. Since 1956, Dr. Berfenstam has devoted himself to social medicine, in which discipline he became professor in 1960 and, in 1961, professor and chairman, Department of Social Medicine, University of Uppsala. Over the years, Dr. Berfenstam has been engaged in research into many aspects of social medicine, including biochemistry, preventive medicine, and medical-care problems, especially international comparisons of the consumption of and the need for medical care. A consultant to the World Health Organization on several occasions, he serves as a consultant to national civic and health-care institutions in Sweden.

Thomas W. Bice is professor of health services and a member of the Health Services Research Center of the Department of Health Services in the School of Public Health and Community Medicine of the University of Washington. He is also the director of the Health Policy Analysis Program, a unit within the School of Public Health and Community Medicine that executes analyses of health issues for the state legislature and its Department of Social and Health Services and Hospital Commission.

Stuart S. Blume, senior research fellow, Department of Sociology and Psychology, Chelsea College, University of London, received the Ph.D. from Oxford University in 1967. Thereafter he was employed by the Science Policy Research Unit, University of Sussex, the Department of

Education and Science, the Organization for Economic Cooperation and Development, the Civil Service College London, Institut d'histoire et de sociopolitique des sciences, Université de Montréal, and the Cabinet Office, London. In addition to his research responsibilities at the University of London, Dr. Blume serves as research secretary to a Working Group on "Class Inequalities in Health," the Department of Health and Social Security Chief Scientist's Organization, recorder of the sociology section of the British Association for the Advancement of Sciences, and consultant to the Organization for Economic Cooperation and Development. He is the author of *Toward a Political Sociology of Science* and the editor of *Perspectives in the Sociology of Science,* among other publications.

R. G. S. Brown, director of the Institute for Health Studies, University of Hull, at the time of his death in June 1978, received the Ph.D. from the University of Hull in 1972. Joining the National Service in 1951, he served as assistant principal, Ministry of Health and Local Government (Northern Ireland), tutor to postgraduate hospital administrators training scheme, lecturer in social administration, University of Manchester, principal, Scottish Home and Health Department, lecturer, senior lecturer in social administration, the University of Hull, consultant to the SSRC on management in the public sector, external examiner at Manchester, Strathclyde, UCNW, and Glasgow College of Technology. His principal publications include *Reorganising the Health Service, The Management of Welfare,* and *The Administrative Process in Britain.*

W. Robert Curtis is the president and founder of Social Matrix Research, Inc., a company specializing in organizational development and research in human services. His doctorate in health-services administration follows masters degrees in public health, behavioral sciences, and education.

A. Sakari Härö is the Director of the Department of Planning and Evaluation in the National Board of Health of Finland. He is a D.Med.Sc., graduate of the University of Helsinki, and has been educated in London (DPH) and UCLA. He holds an honorary medical degree from The University of Uppsala, Sweden. His clinical specialties are serobacteriology, dermatology, and tuberculosis. In the 1950s he served as State Inspector of Tuberculosis, and in the 1960s as Chief of the Department of National Health Statistics. He has served in his present position since 1970. He is also a member of the WHO Expert Panel on Health Statistics.

John C. M. Hattinga-Verschure, professor in hospital sciences, the medical faculty of Utrecht National University, received his doctorate in chemistry and medicine. After specializing in and practicing internal medicine for twelve years, Dr. Hattinga-Verschure became the medical director of St. Mary's and St. Luke's hospitals in Amsterdam—positions that he served in for ten years. His research is primarily directed toward innovation of care delivery for health.

Jean de Kervasdoué was born in 1944. After a graduate education in France and two years in Africa where he worked as an agricultural engineer, he went to Cornell University. He graduated with an M.B.A., and received a Ph.D. in 1972. Dr. Kervasdoué came back to France and continued his work on medical research and hospital organization at the Centre de Recherche en Gestion of the Ecole Polytechnique. Since then, he has published several articles in the fields of sociology of science, sociology of organization and political economy. For four years, he has also been in charge of economic planning at the agency running Paris University Hospitals. While still doing research and teaching, Dr. Kervasdoué is presently the head of the long range planning unit in the private office of the Minister of Agriculture in Paris.

Rudolf Klein is professor of social policy and administration at the University of Bath. He was home affairs editor and chief leader writer of *The Observer* and senior fellow at the Centre for Studies in Social Policy. His main research interests are public expenditure and health politics. Among his many publications are "Ideology, Class and the National Health Service," *Complaints Against Doctors, The Politics of Consumer Representation* (with Janet Lewis), and *Inflation and Priorities.* Dr. Klein is writing a book on *The Politics of Health, 1946 to 1976,* an analysis of the first thirty years of the British National Health Service.

Jean François Lacronique graduated from the school of medicine at the University of Paris in 1970. After one year of training at IBM France, he was appointed to the Ministry of Health, where he was in charge of developing policy for the use of computers in the field of medicine. In 1973, he was sent to the United States to serve as Science Attaché at the French embassy in Boston, and in 1977, he graduated from the Sloan School of Management at M.I.T. Dr. Lacronique became medical editor of *Le Monde* upon his return to France in 1978; more recently, he was appointed director of the Direction Générale de la Santé et des Hôpitaux, one of the three major branches of the French Ministry of Health and Social Security.

Theodore R. Marmor, professor of political science and public health at Yale University and chairman of the university's Center for Health Studies, received the Ph.D. from Harvard University. He was formerly associate professor, School of Social Service Administration, and research associate, Center for Health Administration Studies, University of Chicago. The author of *Politics of Medicare* and the editor of *Poverty Policy,* his most recent publication on the politics of health, welfare, and social security includes *Political Science and Health Services Administration* (with Andrew Dunham).

James A. Morone is a research fellow at the University of Chicago Law School and a doctoral candidate in political science. His dissertation centers on efforts to represent consumers on public-planning boards. He has written numerous articles on health politics and policy in the United States.

Frieder Naschold is Director of the International Institute for Comparative Social Research of the Science Center Berlin. He was formerly professor of political science at the University of Constance and was elected president in 1974. Previously Frieder Naschold was visiting professor at Harvard University and the Institut für Höhere Studien in Vienna.

Duncan Neuhauser is associate professor of health services administration at the Harvard School of Public Health in Boston, Massachusetts. His doctorate in business administration is from the University of Chicago. His research interests are hospital and health care organization as related to costs and the quality of services provided.

Ragnhild Placht received both M.A. and M.S. degrees in psychology. She has been a research assistant in the Department of Social Medicine at the University of Uppsala since 1976.

Simone Sandier took a degree in mathematics and statistics at the University of Paris and has been director of research in the Division of Medical Economics at CREDOC (Research Center for the Study of Observation of Living Conditions) since 1963. Mme. Sandier is active in various committees and councils and has been a consultant for the European Economic Community, the International Labor Organization, and the World Health Organization, particularly in fields connected with health costs and health statistics. She is the author of numerous articles, including "L'évolution des coûts hospitaliers: hôpitaux publics," "La consommation de soins médicaux dans le cadre de l'Assurance Maladie du Régime Général de Sécurité Sociale, évolution 1959–1978," "La démographie médicale dans les pays occidentaux," and "L'évolution des soins médicaux en France: tendances et problèmes."